Managing Health Systems in Developing Areas

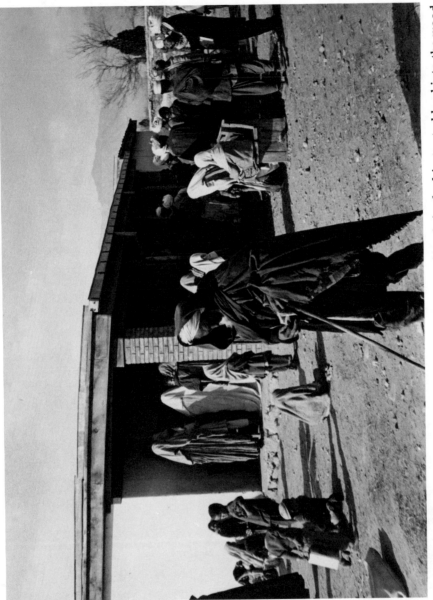

Patients at a Basic Center. The women, completely covered by their *chadris*, try to blend into the woodwork in order not to be noticed by the men.

Managing Health Systems in Developing Areas

Experiences from Afghanistan

Edited by
Ronald W. O'Connor
Management Sciences for
Health

LexingtonBooks
D.C. Heath and Company
Lexington, Massachusetts
Toronto

*To Dr. M.A. Wahabzadha, whose
unswerving dedication to his country's health
made many things possible.*

To the Afghan people, who will prevail.

*And to Grace, Terry, Dick, Ernst, and
Steve, who made all the difference at
the beginning.*

Library of Congress Cataloging in Publication Data

Main entry under title:

Managing health systems in developing areas.

Bibliography: p.
1. Rural health services—Afghanistan. 2. Medical assistance, American—Afghanistan. 3. Underdeveloped areas—Community health services. I. O'Connor, Ronald W. [DNLM: Health services—Organization and administration—Afghanistan. 2. Rural health—Afghanistan. 3. Developing countries. WA395 M266]

RA771.7.A3M36   362.1'068   79–48060
ISBN 0–669–03646–3

Published simultaneously in Canada

Printed in the United States of America

International Standard Book Number: 0–669–03646–3

Library of Congress Catalog Card Number: 79–48060

Contents

List of Figures

List of Tables

Preface

The Management Sciences for Health (MSH) Perspective
Ronald W. O'Connor

More than a decade ago, now-forgotten Afghan and expatriate workers were developing small health posts and programs for rural areas. Nine years ago in the Hazarajat, the mountainous central core of Afghanistan cut off by snow five months of the year, Afghans and expatriate nurses were training illiterate village women to be health workers for their own valleys, well before the international embrace of the primary-care, health-by-the-people credo. This experience was written up, but is almost unavailable today. Eight years ago, on the edge of the plain of central Asia, north of the Hindu Kush, an anthropology team observed village health needs, activities and pathways to care, though the record of their experience is also almost unavailable today.

Seven years ago, a technical-assistance team from Management Sciences for Health (MSH) began working with the Afghan government to improve rural access to health care. Together, the Ministry of Health and the team made some progress and fewer mistakes than they otherwise would have, had they not been able to stand on the shoulders of those who had gone before. The chance exposure to the experience of earlier workers made clear how fragile the thread of continuity could be. This book has been written to minimize the risk that those who carry on with rural health development will inadvertently make the same mistakes yet again.

One of the basic tenets of our philosophy of management assistance for developing-country health programs is that MSH must work for, and through, host-country health decision makers who retain the authority and responsibility for their programs. A result of this belief is that we do not, in general, publish or publicly communicate regarding the programs we serve without the involvement, approval, and usually coauthorship of our host colleagues.

This policy is violated here for two reasons. First, the current political situation in Afghanistan makes it inopportune for former Ministry of Public Health colleagues or current officials to assist in case their actions would be misinterpreted. Second, the passage of time will scatter the data and people beyond practical recall if a summary record of the important lessons learned is not promptly assembled. We therefore offer this book with a mixture of gratitude and regret—gratitude to the country and people for the opportunity to work together, and regret that those involved in Afghanistan who made the important decisions and shouldered the responsibility are not able to be recognized.

The Donor-Program-Manager Perspective
Stephen C. Thomas, USAID Health Program Manager

This book sets forth the experience of the MSH advisory teams that worked within the Ministry of Health in Kabul for nearly 6 years. It represents the combined observations of nine persons who were resident in Kabul as well as various short-term staff members who came to Afghanistan for specific tasks. These nine individuals represented two teams: the first group arrived in mid-1973 and were replaced by a second group of five in 1976. Both groups proved to be diligent, culturally sensitive workers. They were experimenters in the best sense, and they pursued the goal of an affordable, functional health-care-delivery system to the bitter end.

It is important to add a few observations here relating to this MSH/USAID experience within the Ministry of Public Health. The AID method of providing assistance involves the development and funding of "projects" both large and small. Project development places a premium on having competent technicians as designers who understand the country's strengths and weaknesses, are gifted with foresight, and can work with their host-country colleagues. It is obvious that this ideal is rarely attained, particularly in areas as complex as health services. Since project design is frequently imperfect, it is left to those who put the projects into the field to attempt to keep the project headed in the intended direction. In the present era, this duty is delegated to the contract team, with, at most, a project manager in the AID mission. It is on the contract team that the burden of project implementation falls. This team finds the flaws in project design; it finds the targets of opportunity; and it learns what works and what does not. This role leads to development of a unique relationship between the contract team and the AID project manager. To the project manager falls the job of deciding how far to allow the project to deviate from the original design. With project design imperfect, foresight scarce, and perfect knowledge unavailable, a very flexible team and project-manager relationship is required in working toward the same goal. The project manager must be technically competent and willing to accept the responsibility for decisions that allow the project to deviate from its design path but that lead toward the stated goal.

All projects have budgets, and flexibility in the use of funds is limited. Frequently, as projects develop, experimental opportunities arise that were never foreseen. Usually, the limiting factor is funding. Every project should have a fund available for discretionary use by the project manager to fund unforeseen opportunities. Much can be accomplished at times with just a few thousand dollars.

We are frequently asked whether this was a "successful" project. How does one define success? In the sense that the MSH team defined the management problems in the Ministry, showed how the Basic Health Center could be made to operate more effectively, devised two alternative health-care-delivery systems, and trained the workers and set them in the field, this project was a success; a body of knowledge and experience has been accumulated that can be drawn on. In the sense that we did not leave behind a functioning system serving all rural Afghanistan and managed by a competent Ministry, the project was a failure. However, the political events so common in the past 20 years can conspire to defeat the best efforts. It is essential that any country have political stability before much can be accomplished.

Finally, a word of appreciation and thanks to the three groups of people:

The MSH organization and its teams, who were a pleasure to work with.

Those AID personnel, both in Kabul and Washington, who were interested and supportive.

The Afghans in the Ministry who allowed participation in the development of their health-care-delivery system. They have been the real victims of the events of the last 2 years.

Acknowledgments

The Ministers and Ministry staff for whom we worked cannot currently be acknowledged, yet they bore the responsibility and made the project possible. Under normal circumstances, they would be coauthors.

The project was fortunate to be guided by enthusiastic and perceptive donor representatives: from USAID, Grace Langley catalyzed the whole process by her effective groundbreaking with the Ministry as health/population officer; Charles Gurney carried the project through the middle years; and Steve Thomas had the job of winding it up when the political situation deteriorated. Vince Brown and Chuck Grader were constantly supportive as mission directors. In Washington, the path was smoothed by Barbara Turner, John Alden, and Allen Randlov in the NENA Bureau, and by Gladys Frazier, Lou Stamberg, Ann Demarel, and Roger Carlson on the Afghan Desk. Three members of the U.S. Embassy were particularly valued allies: Ambassador Ted Eliot and Consular Officer David Bloch were constant supporters who made things happen when others could not; Ambassador Adolph Dubs presided at the end and gave his life in the process.

From the international community, UNICEF, through its Resident Representatives Sven Hoelgard and Ted Crunden, deserves particular thanks. UNICEF encouraged the effort every step of the way, materially through support to Basic Health Services and the village programs, and with field staff Paul and Anne Kesterton seconded full-time to the effort. N.N. Beyhum, WHO representative for much of the period, was instrumental in helping to preserve good working relations in the face of pressures that could have easily degenerated into interdonor rivalry, and Ray Manning carried on in the same vein. The U.N. Fund for Population Activities began to make important contributions through the work of Representatives Ted Nelson and Siri Melchior, who picked up substantial commitments to the *Dai* Training Program.

The experience of many others was freely offered and absorbed with great benefit: the University of California/Santa Cruz team supporting the Auxiliary Nurse Midwife School were valued colleagues throughout the project; the Medical Assistance Program (MAP), through the fieldwork of Jean and Rex Blumhagen and Pat Wakeham, kindled the village-worker idea; Louis and Nancy Dupree and Byron and Mary Jo Good gave us added insight into village life. Care Medico's work with Kabul hospitals and Save-the-Children (U.K.) with the Shewaki Center provided clinical training experiences and useful feedback throughout the period.

Peg Hume aided substantially in the process of pulling together project materials, with Pat McCarthy and Marguerite Smit preparing the manuscript. Finally, this report exists because of the encouragement and support of Barbara Pillsbury and Allen Randlov, who found a way to see that some of the lessons learned would be recorded.

This project was funded primarily by The Agency for International Development, under contract AID/PHA c-1037, with important contributions by UNICEF, the U.N. Fund for Population Activities, and MSH.

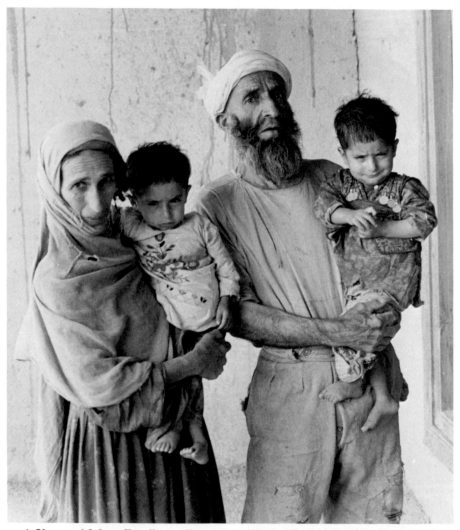

A Young Afghan Family en Route to a Basic Health Center. Their pride and independent spirit are characteristics of the Afghan people.

1

Overview

Ronald W. O'Connor

The Entry Environment

The King is deposed in a coup in July 1973. The new Republican Government of Afghanistan affirms it will honor prior international agreements and, in August, three technicians arrive in the Ministry of Public Health to begin work on one minor element among these agreements.

An elderly clinician without prior public health or management background becomes Minister of Public Health. Exploring his Ministry, he finds that field activities are largely confined to mass smallpox immunization and malaria control. The rural health centers function sporadically as distribution outposts for dried milk, flour, and oil provided through the U.N. World Food Program. Assorted foreign-assistance programs focus on individual hospitals, model clinics, or small geographic areas in an attempt to make some visible contribution. A WHO contingent of eighteen advisors is scattered across the ministry, half focused on the immunization and malaria mass campaigns, with the others diffused, largely without resources, in various Ministry offices. No clear picture of Ministry personnel exists, except as represented by the stream of discontented doctors waiting at the Minister's door who wish they were posted someplace else. The only certainty in the supply situation is shortages. No one seems to know what is available, where supplies are, or who is authorized to move them from the assortment of decrepit storehouses in Kabul. A new warehouse is under construction with AID assistance, bringing hopes that the "poor relation" syndrome and disorganization resulting from years' accumulations of drugs (odd lots, overruns, and expiring drugs and company donations), equipment ("servicable," broken, parts missing, 110 volts only), and medical literature (JAMA, October, 1963, Archives of Orthopsychiatry) may finally be altered.

With disarray of the government health system and new leadership, the majority of Ministry workers seem to be either lying low, hoping to remain inconspicuous, or jockeying for position as the power structure begins to coalesce. Even the ambitious know that it is too early to stake out territory.

Oblivious to this government fluidity, the people continue to seek health care, using the free services of the government system where they can find them, but largely relying on resources in the villages and the towns that make up the private health-care system. Preoccupied with establishing relationships and control in the Ministry, few officials have time to consider promising examples of innovation that may cast light on future trends in Afghan rural health development.

1

A. Introduction

Like layers of successive civilizations in an archeological dig, the developing world is littered with the residue of well-intended national and international efforts to promote health. Enmeshed in a complex of cultural and economic forces, health problems, however, have rarely lent themselves to simple solutions. On a national scale in less-developed countries (LDCs), an attack on health problems in general is often largely a grandiose but ineffectual gesture. In the face of this complexity, pilot health projects with a research focus or demonstration projects on a slightly larger scale operated with intensive resource inputs have become relatively well-known and popular compromises. However, the gap between the pure culture of the experimental model and the political and economic realities of national health implementation is immense, and rarely bridged.

This account of work in Afghanistan reviews attempts to *directly assist in the improvement of a national rural health-care system* over a 6-year period. A resident team of four to five persons worked directly with Afghan health officials throughout the 6 years. This overview includes summaries of where the Afghan health system was, the strategies attempted to improve it, what worked, what failed, and why. The purpose is not to focus on Afghan project history, but to convey essential lessons learned in a productive government-donor relationship focused on management of national-level rural health expansion.

B. Major Findings

Several major findings surfaced consistently throughout the period and formed the practical premises on which the effort was based. These findings are noted here in three categories: development of rural projects, political lessons, and technical assistance.

Development of Rural Projects

"Pilot" projects should be part of a phased commitment to a national program. Independent experimental projects usually cannot be replicated because they tend to enlist people, incentives, and resources unavailable on a national scale, and because they lack the political constituency required for national adoption.

The important constraints in developing village-level health programs are the management support systems for supply and supervision. Initial training is an easier task.

Rural health programs can be designed to be largely self-supporting; villagers commonly spend substantial amounts seeking health care, and they are willing to pay for effective drugs. Prepackaged drugs in course of treatment units with pictorial and written instructions can be sold inexpensively at the village level to make the program financially self-sufficient.

Indigenous practitioners, such as village midwives, can have their skills upgraded by government training programs and can continue to work in their villages in the traditional manner, avoiding complex support systems and government bureaucracy.

Village-level workers (as well as health center workers) need incentives to provide anything other than curative care; these incentives for preventive and health-education work are very difficult to achieve in practice.

Political Lessons

The primacy of decisions based on political reality. Decisions and direction of nationally supported health activities must be expected to mirror the dominant political interest. Data and scientific analyses are, in practice, primarily valued to substantiate the program desired. They are of secondary use for technicians to build cases for alternative strategies, which then may gradually infiltrate program thinking. Projects must recognize that ministry leaders, as well as most donors, have a limited time perspective and need to demonstrate results in terms of 1- or 2-year time horizons. They cannot generally stake their reputations on long-term possibilities alone. The political maxim "what have you done for me lately" is as true in health as in any other field.

Government must appear to serve all the people. Experiments and demonstration projects divorced from a government commitment to extend the experience nationwide are likely to *remain* only experiments for extended periods. Many examples of pilot projects, usually research focused, that were operated with intensive resource inputs are relatively well known in the international health arena; Danfa, Narangwal, and Lampang are examples. Few have graduated to national implementation, and there is only scattered documentation available on the problems and processes of large-scale rural health development.

Local support for village health programs is strong once the benefits are observed. Village committees and local support groups may become helpful only when they are completely convinced that the central government will not or cannot provide support instead.

Ethnic or regional differences within a country do not necessarily mean that separate village programs need to be planned for each group. Demand for health services is widespread, despite differing forms of indigenous health practices.

Technical Assistance

A technician team is much more likely to be effective when it works directly in a Ministry of Health, sharing space and day-to-day experiences with counterparts, as compared with work from a separate location.

A technician team must demonstrate that its loyalty is to the goals and objectives of the Ministry it serves, and not primarily to a funding agency.

Team positioning is important, and access to decision makers essential, because good work and ideas rarely survive by themselves. To move a program, ready access to the centers of power is required.

Credibility with top Ministry officials is a necessary precondition for impact, and it comes in part from helping to "deliver the goods." Ministers and managers often face problems beyond the scope of project workplans. An inability or unwillingness to respond in these ad hoc situations will limit the interest of decision makers in utilizing technical assistance in the future.

Effective management support of a developing country health program requires long-term commitments and relationships. The quick fix is a rare event, and short-term consultants cannot be expected to solve many problems. Management support for decision makers implies establishing relationships of trust, credibility, and shared commitment which the short-timer cannot develop.

C. The Project in the International Health Context

The international health scene in the fifties and sixties saw the rise of vertical, disease-specific programs for smallpox and malaria, followed by increased attention to the fixed, multipurpose health-center concept in the late sixties and early seventies and the subsequent rise to prominence of village-level or "primary-care" efforts.

This project paralleled early phases of the shift in world interest toward expansion of access to primary care for the rural majority. The project stemmed from a Minister's concern that the development of basic health services was beset by great disparities between public expectation and Ministry performance in the practical management of rural health delivery.

The Minister's explorations with donors and USAID's placement of the first health/population program officer in Kabul led to development of a project proposal focused on rural family health services. Two major elements were envisioned: a *training program for female auxiliary nurses* to begin to fill the maternal and child-care vacuum in a Moslem society with a health system staffed by males, and a *rural health-management development program* described here.

The central objective of the project was to assist with the implementation of rural health-service systems, which implied living within the constraints of available knowledge; of personnel working under government procedures, regulations, and incentive systems; of sustainable budget limits and vagaries of a constantly varying political climate in which Ministry decision makers resided.

The first two and one-half years of the project involved initial situation analysis, building relationships by working with the existing Basic Health Center system, and assessing the potential of alternative and complementary health-service mechanisms that might be used to reach the majority of the population beyond the scope of formal government systems. The second stage added the testing and implementation of village-based delivery systems potentially able to reach this remote rural majority.

Government-sponsored rural health systems around the world can be characterized as large organizations with remote, decentralized delivery units. They all employ relatively stable, well-known kinds of health knowledge and technology, where little is unique or specialized to a particular situation. These organizations are concerned with the individual as well as collective good; they are faced with constantly rising and unachievable public expectations; they are often operated on the premise that nobody should be denied service (whether or not they or the government can pay); they are enmeshed in the rules and procedures of civil service and government bureaucracy; they are staffed by technicians, professionals, and social workers usually without experience or training in the practical management tasks that form the bulk of their work—in short, they must be among the most frustrating and challenging of work environments. The message of this book is simply that given host-country commitment, progress can be made—even in the most difficult environment—in the practical delivery of rural health services in a developing world.

D. Organization of the Book

This chapter concludes with a chronology of events to aid in keeping the evolution of project activities in perspective and a summary of the initial entry process. Chapter 2 examines the Basic Health Center system and the actions taken to improve it. Chapter 3 summarizes the development of alternative delivery systems—village health workers and *dais*—for village health services. Chapter 4 looks at the central-management support systems required to serve the rural programs, and chapter 5 discusses the roles and relationships of the host country, the donors, and the technical-assistance contractor. Chapter 6 deals with the interactions of field team and central office in international health-program operation. Chapter 7 includes short discussions of pilot projects, the perennial vertical/horizontal program debate, and observations on local management style. A separate section of appendixes provides more detail on rural surveys, the indigenous health system, village program development, financial analyses, and a critique of the Basic Health Center idea. A glossary, Afghan/Gregorian calendar conversion, and list of documents are included in the backmatter.

E. Chronology

Figure 1-1 outlines the evolution of events and activities during the project. Major political events—coups and changes in Ministers—are noted along the time scale on the left. *Central-ministry management-support activities* are noted on the right margin, and the major field activities—*basic health services* and the development of *alternative delivery systems*—are summarized in the center of the figure. A chronology of dates and events is included at the end of the book.

F. Organizing the Technical-Assistance Program: Initial Entry and Problem Analysis

The team arrived in Kabul under rather fluid circumstances. Within the Ministry the reception was warm, but officials had no clear expectations for the team in context of the government change and were preoccupied with their own positioning. Their prior experience with technical assistance and foreign advisors, while not without occasional bright spots, had been generally unexciting. There was no reason to think that this situation might be different or to invest much energy for a very speculative return.

The start-up was slow. Where to put them? Counterparts? A telephone? A positive aspect of the major change in government was that there was no immutable commitment by the Ministry to the status quo. Difficulties and problems could readily be attributed to leadership no longer present, without personal identification or responsibility, which eased the process of initial analysis of Ministry systems and procedures that impacted on rural health.

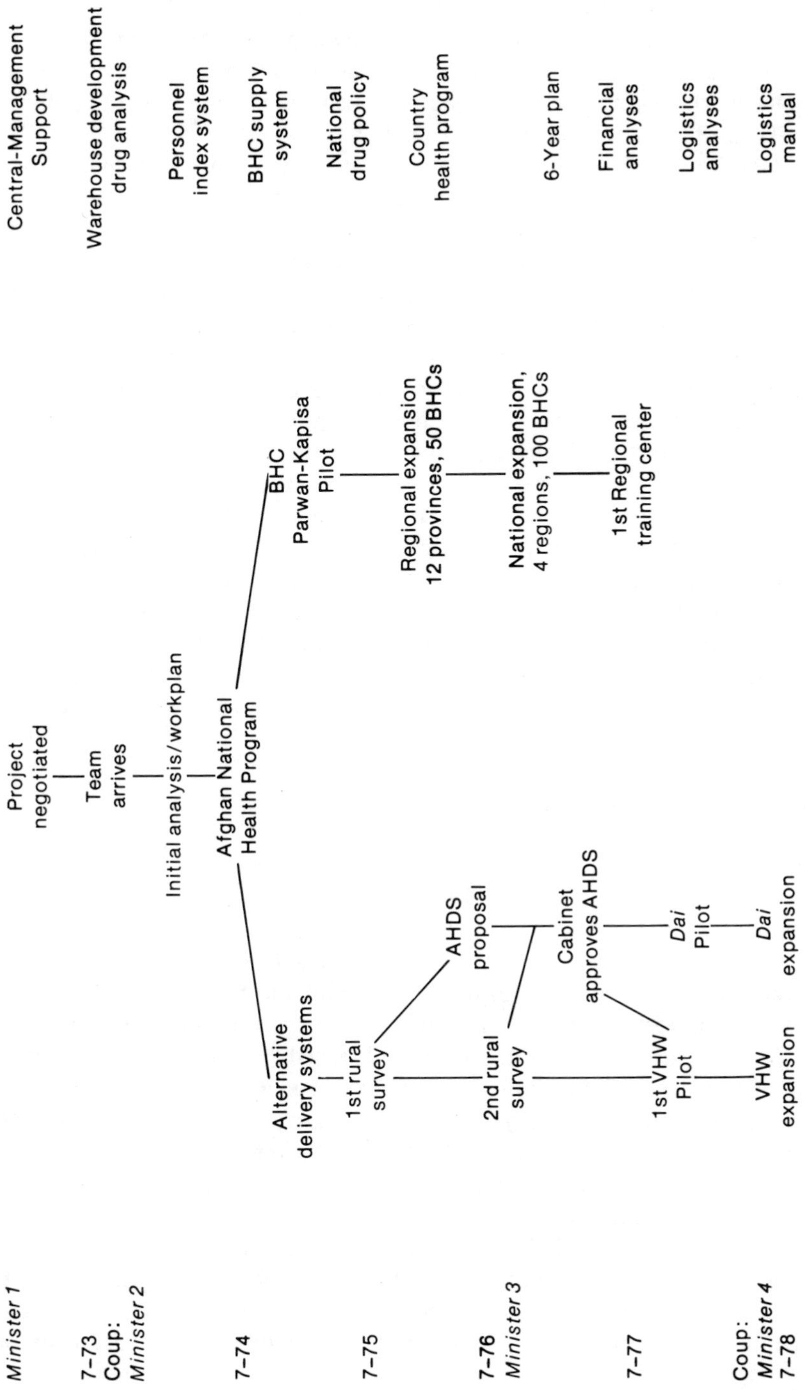

Figure 1-1. Project Evolution

The first steps by the team were important and would surely be observed and evaluated as indicators of management-team prospects. A two-part approach was used, with equal attention to some concrete steps toward working with the Ministry on problem solution and to the building of relationships with Ministry personnel.

Despite the disarray brought on by the change in government, there were still obvious problem areas that concerned the Minister and that most staff members could agree were bottlenecks. Basic Health Services was one, the focus of the initial agreement between the Ministry and AID. Two others were the warehouse and supply system and the procurement and use of pharmaceuticals. Both were selected for immediate attention in the start-up phase of the project for several reasons: they were immediate, widely perceived needs within the Ministry; they were significant problems that were not on the way to solution, yet might respond to technical assistance in a relatively short time frame and in a visible way; and they would demonstrate the team's commitment to assisting the Ministry solve problems of immediate concern rather than focusing primarily on long-range glamour issues. The latter were of interest, of course, but they simply had limited place in an initial strategy aimed at building relationships around mutual and immediate needs: the team's need to demonstrate credibility, technical competence, and position with a broad range of Ministry staff; the Minister's need to demonstrate control and movement of the Ministry; and Ministry staff members needs for position with their peers and the Minister.

Developing the Workplan

The long-range project purpose was to improve rural health services. The only major mechanism specified by the Ministry and AID agreement was the use of Basic Health Services as a means to that end. The work strategy the team employed throughout the project would be a two-part blend of *current-operations support* for day-to-day Ministry functions and *forward-planning* support to help define new directions. In the initial 6 months of the project, current-operations support focused on start-up and organization of a new central warehouse and on drug procurement and use. Forward planning was the initial analysis itself, exploring and documenting Ministry operations as a precondition for rural health-systems improvement. Figure 1-2 depicts the bifocal approach to current operations and forward planning used throughout the project.

The warehouse/logistics problem was an appropriate and continuing concern throughout the project, a symbol of the undramatic, essential, often neglected support systems on which the entire Ministry's impact depended. Construction of a new central warehouse provided an oppor-

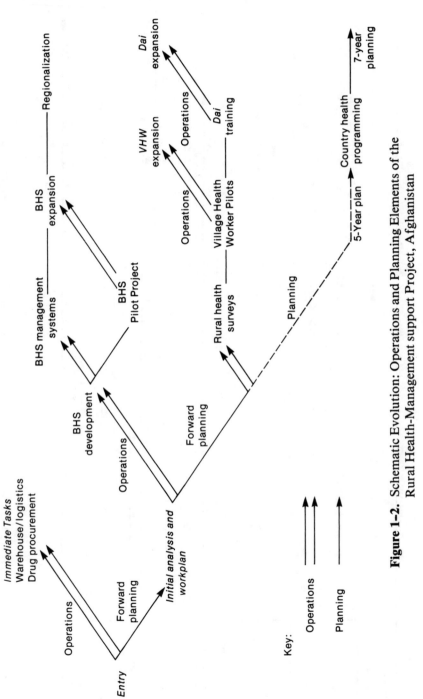

Figure 1–2. Schematic Evolution: Operations and Planning Elements of the Rural Health-Management support Project, Afghanistan

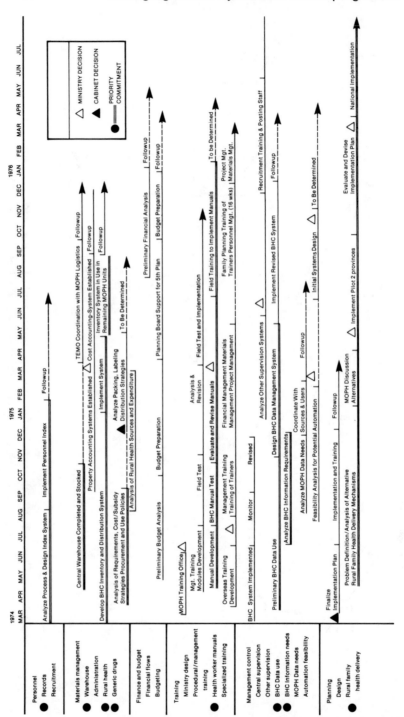

Figure 1-3. Management Support for Rural and Family Health, Afghanistan

tunity to rethink and to implement new organization, procedures, and staffing patterns. Drug procurement provided a similar kind of opportunity to work through a technical problem with leaders of the medical community—what drugs, in what forms, will be obtained by what procedures for Afghanistan? Both these topics are explored later.

With the initial analysis in hand, the Minister, his senior staff, and the team examined the array of constraints on rural health development that might be attacked and rated them in light of four criteria:

1. *Need*
2. *Ministry readiness* to act
3. *Capacity* of Ministry and allied resources to deal with the problem
4. *Leverage,* or relative payoff, in rural health-services improvement anticipated from successful resolution

From this combination of political and technical judgment emerged the workplan, figure 1-3, which focused on (1) Basic Health Services expansion, and (2) Central Ministry planning and analysis of alternative and complementary approaches to rural health.

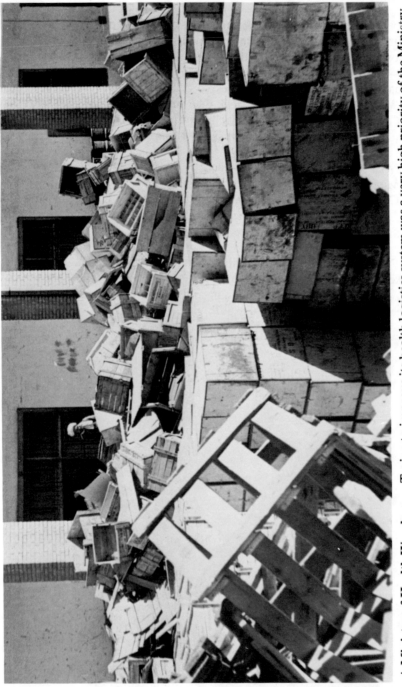

A Ministry of Health Warehouse. Trying to improve its health logistics system was a very high priority of the Ministry, including the central warehouses in Kabul.

2

Working with What Exists: The Basic Health Center System

John W. LeSar and
Ronald W. O'Connor

A Minister's Day

At 8:00 A.M., a queue of petitioners waits on the stair outside the office: the waiting room is full of officials and a couple of well-dressed foreigners; a hospital director wants supplies unavailable in the country; a doctor separated from his family by his posting pleads for transfer; a visiting foundation official, in the country only 2 days, wishes to present his organization's view of the world and potential offerings; the Deputy Minister is assigned to chair a planning meeting to review a piece of yet another long-range national health plan being produced at the insistence of a donor/ technical assistance agency; another Minister calls to inquire whether expensive, special-treatment medical exams might be arranged for his father-in-law in Europe or the states, and his wife also has been having hot flashes; the secretary presents an urgent letter reminding of an imminent deadline after which a major assistance project may be lost for another year; a report arrives on a senior official wrecking a Ministry vehicle while inebriated at a party given by a donor representative; a skeptical cabinet awaits a presentation of the new health initiatives; an opening speech is required at a refresher course; an invitation to participate in a major international seminar in Rio, lasting 4 days plus travel (first class, expenses plus honorarium) arrives personally for the Minister; two rival officials politely backstab each other's performance to their old classmate, the Minister; a man with Hodgkin's disease cannot find nor afford the $500 medical treatment that may save his life; a provincial governor phones to complain about a doctor and asks why the new health center is not finished yet after 2 years.

At 7 P.M., a village headman and two military doctors remain in the waiting room; a diplomatic reception is scheduled in a half hour. It is difficult to be impolite....

A. Overview

Basic Health Centers (BHCs) had evolved slowly through the sixties to a point in 1973 at the beginning of this project where ninety-five BHCs were listed by the Ministry as being in operation. One professional was in charge, and no training capability existed. The BHCs were unmanaged, autonomous medical-care units scattered across the country with many vacant posts and much absenteeism. They offered poor-quality sickness care and little organized maternal or child care. Drug supplies arrived about every 2 years, and the drugs were often inappropriate. They offered no public-health activities at an effective level. Less than 2 percent of the rural people used BHCs in a given year.

The BHC activities were a central and continuing focus throughout the life of this project, and they included several major phases of work; an initial analysis, a pilot project, and a national expansion program initially utilizing centrally managed mobile teams and, later, regional centers for training and support services.

Five years later in mid-1979, with 138 BHCs in operation, the Basic Health Services Department has thirty-five management staff members and fifteen continuing-education trainers. They have considerable skills in planning, scheduling, logistics management, use of information for decision making, and evaluation. The training staff possesses considerable skills in on-the-job training in the field and in teaching methods for didactic presentations. There are operations manuals, continuing-education systems, management-control systems, and drug-supply systems in varying degrees of development and effectiveness. While management and training capacities now exist, most personnel are not yet able to plan, manage, and evaluate activities independently at a reasonable level of effectiveness. They can perform well under supervision, but more supervised experience seems necessary.

Similarly, the improvements in the BHCs themselves are variable. Certain critical problems still remain, particularly in personnel management. Community-health activities now exist only in the form of associated village programs, the VHW and the *dai*. However, drug supplies are improved; the quality of sickness care, maternal care, and child care is modestly improved; and family-planning services are now offered. The average BHC affects less than 8 percent of its service area. Indigenous practitioners and shopkeepers still provide the majority of care outside of the family.

The BHC Department has improved more than most other parts of the Ministry, but it is still not a very effective unit for rural health care, and its role as a community public-health unit is barely visible. Despite these problems, the Basic Health Centers have made relatively large strides over the 6-year period and remain the most visible symbol of rural-government health activity. They are a building block for rural health, surrounded by a demanding environment. They are expected to deal with multiple problems and constituencies with the most rudimentary resources. They may be "basic," but they are not simple (see appendix D), and they must be dealt with in any major program aspiring to attack rural health needs.

Section 2.B describes the baseline status of BHCs in 1973, the changes made over the ensuing 6 years, and their status in 1979. Section 2.C summarizes the findings and lessons learned in the BHC development process.

B. The Basic Health Center Development Program, 1974–1979

Basic Health Services in 1973, When the Project Began

The Basic Health Services Department (BHSD) in Afghanistan in 1973 could claim ninety-five Basic Health Centers (BHCs) on the inventory and a one-person professional staff in Kabul. The department was situated within the Presidency of Preventive Medicine, so the director was two levels removed from the Minister's office. The Minister at that time, concerned about the status and unrealized potential of the Basic Health Services in rural health, requested assistance from USAID, and that request resulted in this project.

Status of the BHCs in 1973: The objectives of the BHCs were to offer basic medical and public-health services to their surrounding areas. Theoretically, the catchment population was 25,000 people, but in reality, only 1,000 to 1,500 different people might visit a BHC in any given year.

To accomplish its objectives, each BHC was authorized to have the following personnel: one doctor, one trained female health worker, one male nurse, one sanitarian, one vaccinator, one clerk, one storekeeper, and one sweeper. However, BHCs were unpopular assignments. Posts were often vacant, turnover was high, and personnel were often assigned but absent.

In 1973, the BHCs usually had inadequate and unstandardized medical equipment. Drugs were always in short supply, and many were inappropriate for BHC use. Antibiotics, vaccines, and intravenous fluids were often out of stock, so effective emergency care, critical-sickness care, and immunizations were not always available.

The BHC was primarily a medical unit that offered care to sick people. The quality of care was poor, since doctors seldom did physical examinations and often lacked the skills necessary for effective emergency or acute care for common problems. Lab tests were practically never ordered. Thus a sick patient who came to a BHC would have a short history taken and the doctor would prescribe drugs without further workup. A visit would take about a minute. The BHC was usually unable to offer much service for minor surgical problems, sprains or fractures, or gynecological or mental problems.

Maternal care was practically nonexistent. Pregnant women seldom came to a BHC because trained female health workers were not in place at many BHCs and the women were reticent to come to male personnel. When prenatal services were offered, they were usually of poor quality. The BHCs did not offer family-planning services, nor special care for lactating women. Women were mostly attracted to BHCs by the distribution of free food through the World Food Program.

Child care also was poor. Immunizations were done sporadically, and no assessment of growth and development (including nutritional assessment), vision, or hearing was done.

As a result, the BHCs provided medical services to ten to twenty patients per day. Of the patients, most were men who visited for relatively minor complaints. Only half the visits were by women and children, although they comprised 75 percent of the population.

Besides care at the BHC, the BHC was supposed to provide some outreach services to the community of a public-health nature. Except for sporadic and unplanned immunizations and facilities inspections, the BHC did not perform these services. There were no effective surveillance, community family-planning motivation, school health, safe water, safe latrine and waste disposal, or health-education programs in the community.

Management and administrative functions within the BHC were poorly executed. The doctor was supposed to maintain management control over personnel, but rarely filled out records regularly or controlled the quality of work. The BHC had no control over the order of drugs and supplies, and all BHCs were scheduled to receive the same amount, irrespective of the population they served. It was not unusual for a BHC to receive no drugs or supplies for 2 years.

Basic Health Services Headquarters in 1973. One physician was responsible for continuing education and management of the ninety-five BHCs in the country. He had a public-health degree and was an extremely dedicated man, but he had no experience in any aspect of health-manpower planning or training nor in health-services planning, scheduling, logistics management, information systems, financial management, personnel management, public relations, health-services research and development, or evaluation. His staff consisted of high school graduates who performed clerical tasks. Thus no training or management system existed at the headquarters office.

Other Areas of the Ministry Affecting Department Operations. Few training skills existed within the Ministry in areas pertaining to basic health services. Basic training of paramedical workers such as nurses, sanitarians, and vaccinators was conducted, but the training personnel were not skilled in job analysis, supply-and-demand analysis, curriculum development, student evaluation and testing, or training administration. As a result, inappropriate numbers of personnel were being trained; the training did not directly relate to the jobs at which the workers would be assigned; the training did not guide students through a logical progression and sequence of knowledge and skills; the training was not in BHCs so that the students could experience their jobs under supervision; there was no evaluation; there was no coordination so that changes in the department would result in changes in training; and there was no continuing education. The medical schools were in the Ministry of Higher Education and suffered similar problems. Most new doctors had never visited a BHC at the time of graduation.

The BHC Department was almost totally dependent on the Administration Department for basic support functions pertaining to the BHCs. For example, recruitment and posting of new personnel was handled entirely by the Administration Department on the advice of the Transfer Committee, a committee of senior Ministry officials, of which the Basic Health Services Director was not a member.

Other ministry departments provided limited support for Basic Health Services. The Planning Department had little influence on ministry policy or operations. There was no research-and-development group responsible for testing innovations, nor any evaluation group to assess activities of the BHCs.

With this state of underdevelopment of the BHC management systems, it is not surprising that little was accomplished. A yearly plan was produced, but it merely summarized inputs. There was no supervisory program. The statistical reports were inaccurate, arrived 3 to 6 months late if at all, and were not analyzed in a form to help decision making. Thus decisions were made largely on subjective grounds, since the staff had little experience in using objective data for decision making and little objective data to work with.

Work scheduling was ad hoc, and the department responded to problems—it did not plan to prevent them. The clerks did not know what to do in their jobs, so tea drinking and social conversation were the predominant daily reactions to the anxiety and helplessness that pervaded the office. The director had numerous other responsibilities and was often absent from the department for 3 or 4 hours a day.

The Ministry of Public Health (MOPH) was a traditional ministry, following age-old cultural patterns of management. These patterns caused all decision making to flow to, and await, the highest person available—usually the Minister. He made innumerable daily decisions based on a patron-client system, where petitioners came and presented their cases. He would dispense advice, rules, and policies on the basis of the oral presentations of his petitioners—whether the petitioner was the Deputy Minister, the Director of Basic Health Services, a sweeper in the Ministry, or someone seeking travel permission for health reasons.

The Drug-Supply System: The sporadic provision of drugs to BHCs had roots in the Central Ministry in Kabul. The Administration Department, staffed largely by elder clerks, struggled with a scattering of decrepit storehouses and accountability procedures that favored security over access, hoarding over timely use, and confusion over order. Supplies for BHCs were periodically issued, based on a fixed list that had long been isolated from user feedback. While the list was the basis for shipment planning, in practice shipments were combinations of what could be found in the storehouses and what arrived from UNICEF and other donors. The result at the health centers was several years' supply of some items and inadequate supplies of others, with no mechanism for exchange or sharing with other BHCs.

The Parwan-Kapisa Pilot Project

After the Ministry and the team analyzed the Basic Health System, the Minister pressed for a focused attack on the problems that were limiting BHC performance in both medical and public-health areas as well as in management functions. The question was how to proceed.

During discussions among the Minister, the President of Preventive Medicine, the Director-General of Basic Health Services, and the team in early 1974, the idea for a BHC pilot project took form as a means of evaluating many existing Ministry policies and testing the *practical limits of the BHC system* for providing access to rural health services. By late 1974, a pilot project was underway in six BHCs in Parwan-Kapisa, a province located north of Kabul. Within the project area, a strategy for improvement, consisting of a combination of inputs, was field-tested. This combination was as follows:

Operations Manuals		Frequent Continuing Education		Regular Management Control		Adequate Drugs
Operations		Frequent		Regular		Adequate
Manuals	+	Continuing	+	Management	+	Drugs
		Education		Control		

Operational manuals were developed, based on a job analysis of BHC tasks. Each manual had two major information areas: *technical information* about appropriate medical and public-health activities for the common problems faced at BHCs and *management procedures* for the BHC activities. Manuals were developed for the BHC doctor, the female worker, the male nurse, the sanitarian, and the clerk. The manuals defined "standard packages of care" and "standard management/administrative tasks." Job descriptions, divisions of responsibility, and workplans for all BHC personnel were included. Flowcharts guided workers through the steps of major health problems. A triage, or "filtering," system was developed, where one staff member determined each client's chief complaint and routed him or her directly via a simple color code to the male nurse, the female health worker, or the doctor. Flowcharts guided workers in the steps of each standard package.

Frequent continuing education was a second input in the Parwan-Kapisa project strategy. A team consisting of a doctor, a nurse, a nurse-midwife, and a sanitarian was developed in the BHC headquarters staff. They received training in the contents and use of the manuals for in-service training and became a mobile training unit. Under the supervision of the Ministry and the team, they trained BHC personnel at the six pilot-project sites, working in a counterpart relationship with their colleagues.

Regular management control was a third component, and two approaches to management control were employed: supervision and improved statistical recording and reporting. The trainers also became supervisors, and the concept of the mobile-training/supervisory team was developed. Supervisor checklists were developed for deficiency detection. Registers and reporting procedures at the BHCs were simplified and developed so that recording of data was easy and reports could be generated for headquarters without difficulty.

Adequate drugs was the fourth component of the strategy. A revised list of low-cost generic drugs appropriate for health-center conditions was developed. UNICEF assisted with the procurement, and the drugs were prepackaged in Kabul in "course-of-treatment" units, using sealed plastic bags with color-coded instructions in written and pictorial form inside. The nurse and the female health worker had authorized access to prepackaged drugs for the problems they were trained to deal with, and they referred patients to the doctor only when required.

The level of inputs over the course of the pilot project was at an annual rate of about eight training visits per BHC per year, five supervisory visits per BHC per year, and adequate drugs. The quality of the inputs was high, with team personnel plus other foreign advisors from WHO and UNICEF and senior Ministry doctors all participating. Adequate communications with Kabul and good transportation were obvious assets.

Results: After 9 months of project implementation, there were strong improvement in many of the areas tested, as noted in table 2–1. The Minister was very pleased with the Parwan-Kapisa results, and as word spread through political channels, he immediately pressed for rapid expansion to other parts of the country. However, four inputs had been implemented

Table 2-1
Results from the Parwan-Kapisa Project

Problem Identified in Early 1974	Parwan-Kapisa Results
1. Low utilization of BHCs	Utilization tripled
2. Underrepresentation of women and children under age 5 at BHCs	Slight increases: females 41 to 47 percent, children 20 to 23 percent.
3. Low population coverage by BHCs	Most people using BHC live within 4 miles, so over 75 percent of population is not covered.
4. Poor-quality maternal child services	Strong improvement in pregnancy care at the BHC.
	Demand existed for family planning at the BHC
5. Poor-quality child-care services	Strong improvement in assessment of growth and development using child care
	Moderate improvement in childhood immunizations (50 percent)
6. Poor quality of selected sickness-care problems	Strong improvement in diarrhea care
	Improved diagnosis of malnutrition, but not improved treatment
7. Lack of definition of management/administrative tasks for BHC workers	Worker scheduling implemented
	Patient-flow system implemented

simultaneously: operations manuals, frequent continuing education, regular management control, and adequate drugs. Which input or combination of inputs was most significant? Could diminished levels of inputs lead to performance changes on a national level? Moving from the province of Parwan-Kapisa with six BHCs to the rest of the country with its eighty-nine additional BHCs would surely force a reduction in the mobile-training and supervisory rate. Furthermore, the new personnel brought in for an expansion effort could not be expected to be as highly skilled and motivated as Parwan-Kapisa staff. How much of the success of the pilot project could be replicated across the country? These concerns were important to the team in assessing the results of the Parwan-Kapisa Project.

In addition, the pilot effort had not tested all jobs at the BHC. The BHC purported to offer sickness care, yet skill enhancement in minor surgery, orthopedics, obstetrics/gynecology, and selected critical medical problems such as meningitis or pneumonia care had not been addressed. Community public-health activities were not addressed. It was impossible to test more than a few critical systems in a BHC at a time. Other areas remained for later years.

Thus, at the end of the pilot project in mid-1975, the BHCs in Parwan-Kapisa were much improved, and some systems had been tested for development of national-level BHC training and management support. The project was viewed as a success despite the many areas of uncertainty, and political pressures mounted to rapidly expand the pilot strategy throughout the country.

National Implementation Strategies

Following the pilot project, the Ministry began to apply parts of the Parwan-Kapisa strategy on a wider scale. Three phases can be described: decentralization of management and training to regions through a Twelve-Province Expansion Project, expansion of the mobile-training/supervisory team approach using Kabul-based teams, and the development of regional centers for training and supervision.

The Twelve-Province Expansion: Immediately following the initial results of the Parwan-Kapisa Project, the Ministry began to expand this strategy to forty-one previously unaffected BHCs in twelve provinces, which were divided into four regions centered in Baghlan, Mazar-i-Sharif, Kandahar, and Kabul. Whereas only 5 percent of all operating BHCs were included in the pilot project, the initial expansion would reach 43 percent of the total. The plan was to use the operations manuals (revised and improved based on the Parwan-Kapisa experience), mobile-training/supervisory teams, a decentralized management-organization pattern to improve BHC performance, and the revised drug-supply program.

Many factors prevented this approach from achieving results similar to those in Parwan-Kapisa, particularly staffing, support systems (which are both further examined in section 2.C), and politics. On the political side, decentralization to a regional structure met strong opposition within the ministry from provincial health officers. The provincial health officers were senior doctors who had direct authority over a province and were threatened by the apparent shift of authority implied by the appointment of regional directors. The provincial job was a prized one, with status, patronage, a prominent place on the staff of the governor, and focused access to the Ministry in Kabul. In addition, the regional system did not fit with the usual administrative pattern of the government. Few ministries have regional programs, and there was no regional equivalent to the provincial governor. As a result, the regional directors were initially appointed, but without staff or budget.

Although job-authority statements and operations manuals were developed for the regional directors, explicit authority was not delegated. They were appointed, sent out, and given job responsibilities, but they were not authorized to take corrective actions. They were not given adequate staffs and had to rely on mobile teams from Kabul to implement the mobile-training/supervisory component of the Parwan-Kapisa strategy. As a result, the level of training and supervisory inputs to BHCs in the twelve-province area was low: 1 training visit per BHC per year and 0.9 supervisory visits per BHC per year.

Centrally Managed Mobile-Training/Supervisory Teams: The Ministry staff felt that the Twelve-Province Expansion Project had not adequately tested the Parwan-Kapisa strategy on a national basis. In 1976, the mobile-training/supervisory team approach was reinstituted, with all teams resident in Kabul and traveling to rural BHCs on a planned schedule. A four-phase approach was planned. Phase 1 was a needs assessment. Phase 2 was training based on the needs assessment, using the operations manuals and other training materials in a 5-day in-service workshop at each BHC. Phases 3 and 4 were follow-up supervisory and evaluation visits to assess changes in performance and to conduct other necessary training, particularly in community public-health activities.

Sixty percent of all BHCs were visited in phase 1; 47 percent received phase 2 visits, and 9 percent received phase 3 visits. Two evaluations were carried out to assess the results.

In October of 1976, the operations manuals, a major component of the Parwan-Kapisa strategy, were evaluated. The results were disappointing. BHC personnel across the country could not independently use the manuals at an acceptable level of accuracy. In addition, many could not identify the correct diagnostic criteria or treatment plans for some common, but critical problems. BHC workers could not read the manuals themselves after the 5-day training visit and use the manuals appropriately for the range of topics covered. Something was wrong.

As a result, another evaluation was carried out 4 months later. This evaluation was more extensive and attempted to assess both the status of BHCs and the performance of the mobile-training/supervisory teams. The results showed that the training visits made a difference in the ability of the BHC workers to use the manuals, but that great differences existed between mobile teams in their abilities to communicate information. Many teams were minimally effective—at least in improving BHC skills during one 5-day training visit. Few BHC workers had any previous experience with written materials for their own use, and neither manuals nor training visits alone were adequate. A combination was necessary, including skilled trainers.

During this phase, visits for management-control purposes reached 134 total visits for a supervisory visit per BHC per year rate of 1.25. However, only 61 percent of the BHCs were involved in the supervisory experience. Thirty-nine percent were not visited at all. The scheduling and logistics of training teams covering the entire country from a Kabul base were proving unfeasible for a sustained effort. The drug-supply process was a major improvement, with a new Central Ministry warehouse functioning well enough to get the new standard drug lists issued annually, although not in the prepackaged, course-of-treatment form that had worked so well in the pilot project.

By early 1977, it became obvious that the centrally managed mobile-training/supervisory team approach using the operations manuals as a reference text was not working adequately with the levels of management skills and inputs attainable at that time.

Regional-Center Approach. During 1975, the Twelve-Province Expansion Project had been severely constrained by the decentralization dilemma. However, donors, the team, and the Ministry had concluded that decentralization would be necessary for sufficient numbers of training and supervisory visits to be feasible for most BHCs. As a result, four regional centers were planned in early 1976 and included in the second phase of the USAID health-assistance program. The use of regional centers represented a clear shift in Ministry strategy, offering preservice training to all workers and formal in-service training at an attached BHC for each worker in the region on a twice-yearly basis, and this was supplemented by mobile supervisory visits and a mobile-training visit to those BHCs in critical need of improvement. Owing to frequent shifts in BHC personnel, the concept of a "trained BHC" had proved invalid. Frequent transfers resulted in mixtures of trained and untrained personnel, and the strategy of offering each category of worker two courses per year in addition to preservice orientation seemed more realistic.

In June of 1977, the first regional training center opened in Girishk, a small town in southwestern Afghanistan. Initially, Girishk had few staff members, and they were all unskilled in training. It would take all the Afghan year to improve the numbers and skills of the personnel for the center to become truly functional in the spring of 1978. For this reason, mobile teams from Kabul continued to serve other areas of the country as well as help train the Girishk staff. Even though staff was short in 1977, the Girishk Center, with assistance from Kabul, offered seven teaching courses from 2 to 5 weeks in length. Ninety-two percent of the BHCs in the region received one supervisory visit by the regional-center personnel. In addition, the services at the Girishk BHC improved markedly, and as in the Parwan-Kapisa Project, visits tripled. The people would respond to good services.

Senior Ministry officials visiting Girishk were pleased with the progress made, and in 1978, Girishk was approved for an adequate staffing pattern. To train and manage the twenty-five BHCs in the region, the Ministry assigned a formal training team, a mobile training team, a mobile supervisory team, a strengthened statistical and clerical staff, and a full BHC staff. A regional warehouse for storage and distribution of drug supplies was proposed. However, one month into the new Afghan year, the government of Afghanistan changed through a violent coup d'etat. All ministry programs were thrown into chaos, and by the end of summer in 1978, the regional center began to lose personnel and government commitment. Over the ensuing months, rural security decreased owing to insurgency, and the regional activities of supervision and training dwindled to a halt.

Basic Health Services in 1979, When the Project
Was Suspended

By the time meaningful rural work was suspended, the Basic Health Services Department had grown considerably. The number of BHCs increased by 45 percent, from 95 to 138, by 1979. The number of management and training personnel increased from one to a staff of thirty-five people in management areas and fifteen training personnel in 1979. The department was elevated to a presidency, which increased access to senior decision makers. The BHSD was recognized for better management compared with other areas of the Ministry, and other departments were beginning to adopt some of the management ideas first used in the BHSD. At the time of project suspension, BHSD had the only continuing-education staff for worker-skill maintenance and enhancement.

However, the management of BHCs—decentralized across a vast country with few paved roads, difficult communications, and poorly and inappropriately trained personnel who were neither rewarded nor punished for performance on the job—was extraordinarily difficult.

The Centers Themselves: In 1979, the planned service population of a BHC was still 25,000 people, but, as in 1973, the users of the BHC were 2,000 to 3,000 people mostly living within 4 miles or 40 minutes from the BHC. Access to rural care was broadened because there were more BHCs, but more significantly, because of the primary health-care programs that had developed out of recognition of the limitations of any BHC program.

The authorized personnel situation at the BHCs was similar to that of 1973. As before, vacant posts, absenteeism, and frequent transfers were critical difficulties that had not been overcome. The BHC was still primarily a medical unit offering care at the BHC to sick people who came there. The quality of sickness care was improved, particularly in the care of acute infectious diseases, but BHCs still lacked capability in minor surgery, orthopedic care, and other emergency medical services.

Maternal care was improved tremendously when an auxiliary nurse-midwife (ANM) was present. The ANM had received the most appropriate training of all BHC workers, mostly attributable to the USAID-sponsored technical-advisory and participant-training assistance to the ANM school. BHC doctors were still weak in obstetrics and gynecology, although BHCs were now beginning to offer some family-planning services, even though they did not provide IUD insertions or sterilizations. Women still were attracted to the BHC primarily for food handouts through the World Food Program, but many BHCs were now requiring medical screening of the eligible population of pregnant women and young children.

Child care improved. The auxiliary nurse-midwife was a good child-care worker. She knew how to use the child card to assess growth and development, and she could care for diarrhea and respiratory disease.

Overall utilization rates of the BHCs increased and varied according to local perception of the quality of care provided by the BHC staff under the doctor's leadership. The use of BHCs by women and children increased as health information slowly diffused through the rural population. However, male usage still predominated. The people still preferred pharmacies, shops, and indigenous sources of care as their first source of care outside the home, but the use of BHCs was slowly increasing as quality improved.

Community public-health activities remained practically nonexistent. The BHCs lacked the staff and capability to implement effective community programs, and they perceived their job as primarily sickness care and maternal and child health care at the BHC.

Internal BHC management improved. Register books were kept, and the reporting rate and accuracy was much better than before. The doctor still did not feel comfortable doing administrative tasks.

Considerable improvements were made in the area of drugs at the BHCs. The BHCs now had twice-yearly shipments, whereas in 1973 they usually had one shipment every 2 years. The drug shipments were appropriate in type of drug for BHC usage, and generic drug ordering allowed the Ministry to increase the amounts of drugs given to the BHCs. However, the drug systems still were incapable of regulating the amount of drugs given based on the number of services rendered by BHCs. Busy BHCs still ran out of drugs because they received the same amounts as less-active BHCs. This was particularly unfortunate if the drugs or fluids were in emergency- or critical-care areas. However, drug supplies were now received regularly, and the drugs supplies were relevant to the health problems at hand. Supply timing and quantity were still not triggered by use and demand, but by standard orders from the Ministry.

Basic Health Services Management and Training Capability. With the number of BHSD management and training personnel increasing from one in 1973 to fifty in 1979, (thirty-five in management and fifteen in training), BHSD management and training capability considerably exceeded all other

Ministry programs, with the exception of that for malaria. BHSD had developed considerable experience in planning, scheduling, logistics management, use of information for decision making, and applied health-services evaluation. Afghan personnel had moved from a state of nonawareness about many of these management tools to a point of being able to carry them out with assistance. They now knew what information to ask for, but yet they lacked sufficient skills to function independently.

Training capability was likewise much improved, especially in on-the-job training. Afghan personnel now had considerable training and experience in teaching methods and training administration, especially in field settings. However, they could not, with confidence, conduct job analyses, develop curricula to an acceptable level of quality, develop testing mechanisms, or integrate various training approaches into practical programs.

Other Ministry Areas Affecting Basic Health Services: Three other Ministry activities had substantial impact on BHS: The Planning Department, the Administration Department, and the training institutions. Experiences with the Planning Department, which included Manpower Development, were among the earliest and most consistent failures of the project; these are discussed in appendix F. The status of the Administration Department activities and outcomes is examined in chapter 4.

The project did not encompass work with the basic training institutions, with the exception of the ANM school, which under a separate USAID subproject implemented by the University of California/Santa Cruz established and turned out the first trained female health workers for BHCs. The levels of abilities in those institutions remained woefully under-developed and negatively affected the performance of BHC workers greatly.

Drug supply, the responsibility of the Administration Department, was substantially improved through standardization and limitation of the drug list, more effective procurement (see the following vignette) and storage, utilization of competitive procurement and generic nomenclature, and the procedures of the new Central Ministry warehouse. For BHCs, the entire system could be supplied within a 3- to 8-month period by 1979. However, the Administration Department had not developed the capacity to vary annual requirements by health center, nor to effectively handle requests for additional supplies. Shortages and imbalances remained very real, and logistics support more clearly emerged as the major constraint on the current state of BHC performance.

Drug Procurement

Three successive Afghan governments expressed to the team their concerns for the cost and adequacy of drug procurement. Initial analysis in 1973 indicated that the annual wholesale import cost of pharmaceuticals was equivalent to the total national operating budget of the Ministry of Health. Ninety-nine percent of the drugs were imported as brand-name items from sixty foreign firms, with four firms doing half the business. The fifty leading drugs accounted for 55 percent of the total money expended. While two of the fifty leading drugs were available only as patented drugs, the rest were available generically on the world market.

The Ministry requested that the team assist with the drug-procurement process, with the objective of improving availability of quality drugs at reasonable cost for public-health programs. The national formulary was revised with emphasis on drugs that were effective, safe, and inexpensive; improved bidding and contracting procedures were developed; and generic names were used.

Despite the fact that the total drug market continued to increase and rural people in remote areas continued to indicate that access to modern drugs was their highest health priority, certain representatives of the drug industry felt threatened and reacted vigorously. Advertising and detail men were used to discredit the government's efforts with the public and medical community. Consultants working with the Ministry were "set up" to be caught in compromising positions. Overtures were made, suggesting that the team should work with the Ministry in more appropriate areas. Public broadsides impugning the motivation of the team and alleging profitable connections with particular drug suppliers followed.

The president of the local manufacturing subsidiary of a multibillion dollar European firm requested a meeting with the senior AID representatives and the team. He indicated that we did not understand what was going on, that senior officials in the government were "involved." For the clincher, he indicated to the AID director that their U.S. office would contact appropriate congressmen, and that he "would do whatever was necessary, legal or illegal, to protect his company's interest" in Afghanistan. The AID director thanked him for his candor, assured him that the mission was proceeding carefully and in accord with the Ministry requests to the team, and pointed out that procurement procedures being developed by the Ministry were no different from those already in widespread use in both the United States and Europe.

The Ministry continued its course, the team continued its work, and the firm continued to prosper.

Summary

A great deal of effort was expended over a 6-year period to understand the practical limits of the Basic Health Center system and improve its performance. As the major rural health-services activity (until interest in alternative health-delivery systems began to extend government efforts beyond fixed institutions), BHCs underwent major improvements in the 1973–1979 period. At the same time, they were being recognized as more limited in their direct reach than previous plans had acknowledged; BHCs were taking on new importance as training and referral points for the village programs.

C. Findings from the BHC Development Program

The experience of Ministry personnel and their team colleagues resulted in a series of findings of importance to the development of Basic Health Services in Afghanistan. These findings and recommendations are discussed in the following paragraphs in five categories: drug supply and logistics, incentives, the complexity of Basic Health Services, training for rural work, and lessons in management control. They are listed in approximate order of importance to a health system in Afghanistan's current state of development. The first three are discussed elsewhere and are only restated here for completeness.

Drug Supply and Logistics

Drugs are *perceived* by most health workers and consumers as the essence of effective modern medicine. While often ignored by health decision makers as a rather pedestrian topic, drugs are the most expensive, *controllable* item in the health budget and are the substrate upon which most first-line rural health services are based. To be without drugs means no credibility for providers and no consumers for most health services. Early and sustained attention is merited to drug procurement and use in any rural health system.

Incentives

Financial reward, continuing-education opportunities, prospects for advancement, and recognition by peers are incentives that may help motivate rural health workers over the long run. It is unrealistic to expect sustained good performance under difficult conditions from anyone who is not rewarded for it. Projects that employ unsustainable incentive structures (or none at all) are destined to fail or mislead health decision makers looking for solutions to large-scale rural health problems.

The Complexity of Basic Health Services

The only thing *basic* about such health services is the name, which is usually misleading. The attempt to funnel any number of health- or development-related social services through understaffed, ill-supplied, scantily trained, poorly rewarded, and often forgotten peripheral health centers is predestined for failure on any large scale. Appendix D examines this topic in an illustrative way; the essential point is that workers can be expected to perform only a limited number of tasks up to standard. Health programs face the choice of selecting priority tasks on which limited resources will be focused or pretending to cover all tasks and accomplishing little beyond the disillusionment of workers and clients.

Lessons Learned in Training Rural Health Services Workers

Three major areas will be described: the use of operations manuals, the use of mobile teams, and the development of training capacity.

The Use of Operations Manuals: Basic Health Center Manuals to serve as a reference for all health-center personnel constituted one of the major inputs to the original improvement strategy used in the Parwan-Kapisa Pilot Project. Distributed to each worker, in different editions for different job categories, the manual outlined job descriptions, divisions of responsibility and workplans, and presented clear guidelines for action via flowcharts for the medical/public-health problems and management-administrative functions a given worker was expected to handle.

The manuals, in conjunction with the frequent continuing education at eight visits per year, were learned by the BHC workers involved in the pilot project. However, later evaluation during national expansion was disappointing. Much poorer understanding of the manuals was demonstrated after the 5-day training visit, which was the most that could be sustained on a national scale. What were the reasons for this?

The manuals contained too much material for workers to learn either by reading themselves or in conjunction with 5 days of training. Even the doctors, with many years of previous education, suffered from weak reading skills and lack of familiarity with "textbooks" of this nature. Many other workers had never used written training materials of their own before. The training time was too short and the content was too long.

The difficulties in learning the manuals pointed out the problems of trying to achieve basic skills in a continuing-education setting. It was impossible for workers to learn these manuals to the skills level of independent implementation in short periods of time. Experiences in the Auxiliary Nurse-Midwife School, where the manual became an integral part of the curriculum, demonstrated that students required 5 to 6 months to master the manual in a school environment. Experience suggested that a graduate auxiliary nurse-midwife would require a minimum of 235 hours of instruction or about 39 teaching days to learn the skills to a level of independent implementation. The continuing-education approach to the absorption of large masses of material in a short time was an inadequate strategy.

The Use of Mobile Continuing-Education Teams: Frequent continuing education was an integral part of the Parwan-Kapisa Project, with workers receiving about eight visits per BHC per year on an annualized basis. After Parwan-Kapisa, the training-visit rate could not be maintained at such a high level; three alternative approaches were considered: formal courses in Kabul using specialists in the areas of interest (nutrition, family planning, and so forth); training centers based in the regions offering preservice training, formal courses, and mobile training; and mobile training alone. The first alternative was ruled out because the specialists had no rural experience or were not knowledgeable about how to operate health-services programs. The second alternative was selected, but only became operational 9 months before the change of governments. In effect, mobile training teams became the predominant training mode.

Besides the inadequate training time, three other factors hindered mobile continuing-education team effectiveness. The first was inadequate numbers of training personnel. Two to three times the number of training teams would have been necessary to achieve a level of one training visit per BHC per year, which still would have been insufficient, since the learning time was too short and the personnel transfer rate (often exceeding one transfer per year for doctors, male nurses, and sanitarians) was too high. Figure 2-1 illustrates the average number of training visits that occurred over the life of the project.

A second hindrance to mobile continuing-education team effectiveness was the inadequate skills of the trainers. Those available were experienced at "hands-on" practical on-the-job training, but lacked well-developed training plans and schedules of what to teach. They would often spend considerable time cleaning up BHCs, which was relatively nonthreatening to BHC personnel, but allowed skill development in medical/public-health-management/administrative areas to suffer.

The third hindrance to mobile continuing-education team effectiveness was poor attitudes on the part of some BHC workers. Unfortunately, worker attitudes are usually formed during basic training. The basic training schools, with the exception of the ANM school, did not foster positive attitudes about rural health work and did not train people with rural work in mind. Worker receptivity to training was often marginal, especially that of the BHC doctor, who was the primary opinion leader.

Mobile training can be useful

1. To upgrade existing skills in the work environment

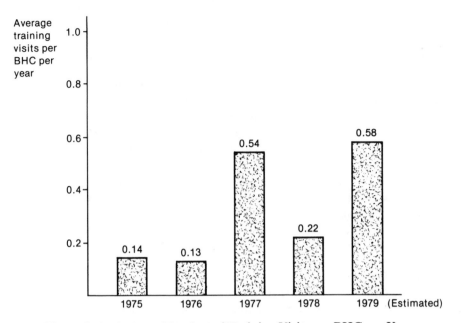

Figure 2–1. Average Number of Training Visits per BHC per Year

2. In conjunction with other training approaches
3. As an aid in recruitment
4. Where length of training is not so long that costs are prohibitive
5. When length of training is not so long or frequent that trainers become discouraged about being away from their normal environment

However, mobile training is a difficult approach for training workers in many new skills, and therefore, it is ineffective as a basic training device. Mobile training is useful in conjunction with other training approaches. The trainers can teach workers in two ways: they can introduce new material to workers through didactic presentations which they can immediately help the workers implement in their own work environments, and they can make on-the-spot corrections of poor or inappropriate work habits based on incomplete understanding of existing skills. Both these advantages are major ones, and observation of the worker in his environment is necessary to plan training programs—whether or not training itself occurs there.

However, many skills can be learned in a fixed training setting where the student's work environment is adequately simulated. For example, to train for BHC work, a training institution can be located at or near BHCs, where the student will work under supervision.

In considering whether or not to utilize a mobile training approach, it is important to list the skills to be taught and divide them into two groups. Group 1 skills can be adequately taught in a fixed institution. These include individual skills for which motivation is not a problem and which students can implement in their work environments without direct supervision. Examples include the application of casts, minor surgical techniques, and medical therapies such as oral rehydration.

Group 2 skills require direct supervision in implementation and hence at least a mobile component. A common situation requiring group 2 skills occurs when workers must work as a team, with each having part of the skills required to complete the task. Common examples are program-development skills: how to plan and implement a community-immunization program, or how to implement a new BHC record or triage system.

An important advantage of mobile teams is *recruitment*. Certainly, in Afghanistan, the *dai* would not travel far from home, and it was necessary for the training to "go to the student." Male village health workers were more comfortable closer to their homes and would more likely travel to a fixed regional training center if one was available.

The *disadvantages* of mobile training include financial costs, which are a result of its low efficiency, and the hardship imposed on the mobile trainers. In Afghanistan, living and teaching in the rural environment is not easy, and accommodations are sparse. The *dai* trainers, being women, had difficulty in traveling beyond their working environments (women in rural areas are mostly restricted to their homes, and the trainers did not want to alienate the village leaders). In these situations, trainer morale suffers when length of training or periods of time away from home become excessive.

The *dai* program, for example, was the longest with 2 to 3 weeks of recruitment and 5 weeks of training. Teacher morale was improved once recruitment was done separately and the teams were in the field for only 5 weeks at a time. In Afghanistan, 4 to 5 weeks at one time and 50 to 60 percent total work time in the field was the maximum tolerable. Personnel performed better and tended to stick with the program if not more than 40 percent of time was spent away from home.

Recommendations for Planning and Implementing Continuing-Education Systems for Rural Health Services: Continuing education can supplement information and skills learned in basic training courses and can prevent decay of skills previously learned. It cannot substitute for inadequate basic training, where inappropriate subject matter is taught and poor attitudes are formed.

Continuing education requires the development of an overall training plan that includes training objectives, planned learning experiences, varieties of training methods, lesson plans, testing, adequate numbers of personnel, and adequately skilled personnel. This may require development of a Continuing-Education Training Unit to which workers are assigned full time.

Students cannot usually use a textbook without being trained with it. Learning the manual requires training courses. If the manual is given without prior training, workers do not understand its contents to a point of independent implementation. Each worker should be trained at least twice yearly. One training session should emphasize subject matter and implementation skills and is best done in groups to share experience. The other training session can be at the BHC, where trainers assist in implementation and observe workers for skill decay.

Workers who share tasks should be trained together. Managers and workers should share common subjects, but have special lessons that help to define their relationships.

Training teams require at least one supervisor for each five teams, and training teams should receive training at least twice yearly with emphasis on improvement of skills in technical areas of training: job analysis, development of training objectives and a training plan, curriculum development (using the objectives and designing learning experiences to serve those objectives), testing, and training administration.

Adequate advisory and consultant time must be planned to develop the basic skills of the trainers. Curriculum development, in particular, is a complex skill. Trainers require about 3 months to learn to perform this skill under supervision. Up to another year of supervised curriculum-development writing, field testing, and revisions is needed before trainers can develop effective curricula independently.

Trainers are specialists and should not be readily transferred to different kinds of work. A Career Development Program should allow trainers vertical career movement in the training field if they perform well.

Developing BHC Management-Control Systems

"Regular management control" was one of the chief elements of the successful strategy used in Parwan-Kapisa to improve BHC performance. All BHCs individually and the system as a whole suffered from poor management: inadequate personnel policies did not reward or punish performance, and inadequate management-support systems within the Basic Health Services and other parts of the Ministry impeded rural health development. A large diverse Ministry with 7,000 personnel existed with an almost total absence of management skills. The following paragraphs discuss experiences in three BHC areas: personnel, supervision, and information systems.

BHC Personnel: The management of BHC personnel was most visible in the continuing and recurring vacancies in BHC posts. These vacancies resulted primarily from two factors: shortages in personnel available and frequent transfers between posts. The transfers signified a general dissatisfaction among workers with living in rural areas; their goal was often to get position closer to Kabul or to their homes and families. Although Ministry rules mandated a 3-year tour before transfer, table 2–2 indicates that this was not enforced.

Much of the absenteeism could be traced to the pursuit of transfers, and workers who came to Kabul would plead their cases before anyone who would listen—even the team, who had no role at all in staff placement. Doctors, male nurses, sanitarians, and lab technicians were fairly successful at this, while the female workers and the vaccinators, coming from the areas in which the BHCs were located, tended to stay there.

What incentives were tried? Free living quarters as an incentive for rural work were gradually acquired, and in 1978, a rural pay differential was developed so that BHC staff in hardship posts received significantly higher pay. Unfortunately, the pay was not related to performance and therefore will not serve as an incentive for good work.

Almost all BHC workers supplemented their incomes through some kind of private service in the medical field. The doctor had a private practice; the male nurse also had some private patients; the female health workers charged for deliveries; and the vaccinators were fee-for-service injectionists in their off hours. Some BHC workers felt that it was not in their interest for large numbers of patients to come to the BHC—it was better if patients came after hours and paid for the service.

Additional incentives in the form of graded continuing-education opportunities are necessary and require more organization and consistency of personnel policies than were feasible at the time.

Supervision in Basic Health Services: Development of supervisory capabilities did continue with personnel receiving on-the-job training; additional personnel were assigned, and three Afghans were sent for management training in the United States in the first year. A regional officers' manual was developed to include supervisory-system objectives and methods.

While this regional element was slow in materializing, supervision for BHCs in the national expansion area had some effects: management/administrative systems that improved within 1 year included worker scheduling, allocation of work among BHC staff, the patient-flow system, doctor supervision, and recording and reporting. Many areas were not addressed, including financial management, personnel management, and coordination of supply and equipment with other parts of the MOPH. The analysis and use of BHC data improved in the first year and then declined; Ministry

Table 2–2
Average Time Posted at BHCs

Position	Average Time Posted (Months)
Doctors	8.3
Male nurses	10.9
Auxiliary nurse-midwives	19.3
Vaccinators	22.6
Sanitarians	9.7
Laboratory technicians	7.2

personnel did not know how to use reports and field data for making decisions. This work was perceived to be tedious and unproductive, and they did not keep it up.

Moving trained supervisory staff from Parwan-Kapisa into the national expansion area precipitated the decline in performance among the initial BHCs. This observation highlighted the problem of inadequate numbers of supervisory personnel. Supervisory visits were never frequent with the continual expansion to BHCs in wider areas. It is clear that the BHCs did not receive regular management attention. As a part of the incentive and career-path plan, many members of the supervisory team staff were scheduled for training in public-health management and were trying desperately to improve their English-language capability through English classes in Kabul. They did not go to the field, but under Ministry rules, they could not be replaced while still in Afghanistan. Consequently, the supervisory visits suffered.

What is the minimum number of supervisory visits per year for effective supervision? Five visits a year achieved significant changes in performance at BHCs in conjunction with continuing education. As an estimate, it would seem that quarterly visits to BHCs should be a minimum input for successful management control.

The mobile teams could do a good job of supervision by following checklists. They made on-the-spot corrections of easily remedied deficiencies, and they wrote reports to the Director of Basic Health Services based on their findings. The supervisory teams were excellent at *finding* deficiencies at the BHCs.

However, once the supervisors returned to Kabul, problems began. Supervisory reports were not structured in an information-giving format, and personnel did not know how to analyze them. Consequently, in most cases, they did nothing. A follow-up system for analysis and action in the Central Ministry was lacking.

As a result of difficulties in correcting deficiencies, it was virtually impossible to maintain a sustained interest in trying to improve the BHCs. In turn, the supervisory teams and the BHCs themselves became skeptical about the Ministry's ability to respond to their needs, with a consequent detrimental effect on motivation and performance. Supervision without mechanisms for remedial action is self-defeating.

Information Systems: As the stock-in-trade of modern managers, information systems were an early and continued component of the project and interest of the team. Whereas special-purpose information-system activities—for example, the rural health surveys and drug-procurement and financial analyses—played a central role in the project, routine information systems did not, with the single exception of supply and logistics. Although considerable effort was expended on the development of routine and annual workplanning procedures, for example, none of them "took." Ministry managers were not accustomed to relying on such information, and decisions were more often made on impressionistic and interpersonal grounds.

While information systems have important roles to play in rural health-services development, priority for their development should be based on potential use, which may well differ from what the outside view might expect.

Recommendations for Planning and Implementing BHC Management-Control Systems:

1. The frequency of supervision visits must be at least quarterly, and at least double the frequency of personnel transfer to have any effect.
2. The ratio of BHCs per full-time supervisory equivalent team should not exceed 20:1 for quarterly supervision.
3. Supervision for deficiencies that cannot be corrected rapidly becomes counterproductive. Delay supervision until at least a minimum number of corrective systems are functioning adequately.
4. In developing new management-control systems, develop *corrective systems at the same time or ahead of* the deficiency-finding systems.
5. If corrective systems are in other departments, ensure coordinating linkages with trained personnel assigned in each department.
6. Develop effective positive and negative incentives based on performance. *Use* the incentives to reward good work and to punish deficiencies caused by poor motivation.
7. Do not punish deficiencies caused by lack of skills. Train these workers instead.
8. If deficiencies *cannot be corrected*, make training visits, not supervisory visits. The BHC is a semiautonomous unit, and programs should

be limited to those which are demanded by the population and which the BHC staff enjoys performing.

9. Expect a 3- to 5-year time period for new management-control systems to be effectively developed.
10. Routine reporting systems may be slow to be used; concentrate on subsystems or procedures that show results quickly to build a positive experience with information systems.
11. Supervisors and consultants should expect to have to do the analysis, make the displays of information, and write the reports for 2 to 3 years until the entire process is routinized.
12. Adequate technical-consultant resources are necessary for all aspects of deficiency finding and deficiency correction in planning management-control systems.

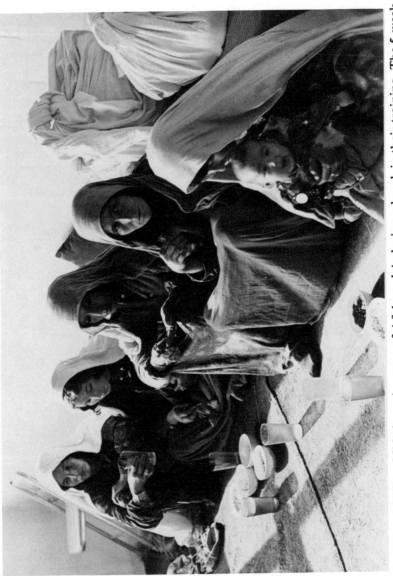

Traditional Village Midwives. A group of Afghan *dais* during a break in their training. The **5-week** course enables them to provide basic services in young-child care, family planning, prenatal care, and hygienic deliveries.

3

Beyond the BHC: Development of Primary-Health-Care Programs

Steven L. Solter,
Peter N. Cross,
and *John W. LeSar*

Village Vignette

Gul Jan was worried this time. His two-year-old son, Ahmad Shah, had never been this sick before; he had a cough that would not quit, a high fever, and a dull, far-away expression so different from his usual happy laugh. Gul Jan's wife, Bibi Khanom, had already tried everything that was available in the village. She had first given her son some old, left-over tablets that she had gotten a year ago for "fever." When that did not seem to help, she had consulted her cousin, an untrained village midwife who had raised seven children. The cousin's advice was to stop giving the child any "cold" foods, especially yoghurt or meat. When Ahmad Shah still failed to improve, she asked Gul Jan to take the boy to Mullah Safruddin in order to get a tawiz, or amulet with holy words from the Koran placed inside. But Ahmad Shah continued to get worse, despite the tawiz.

Gul Jan tried to think of what else he could do. Since it was winter, it would be very difficult to take Ahmad Shah to the nearest doctor at the Basic Health Center in Anderab. Anyway, who could be sure that the doctor had not gone to Kabul or maybe the Health Center was "in-between" assigned doctors. There was always the pharmacy in Anderab, of course, but how much did the pharmacist know about curing cough and fever? If the bus could make it through the snow, he would have to pay 80 Afghani (about $2.00) just for round-trip transportation. If the bus could not get through, that meant 6 to 7 hours trudging through ice and snow with a sick two-year-old.

Meanwhile, Bibi Khanom was trying to comfort the boy and keep him warm. Even though he was thirsty, she felt it was important not to give him too much to drink, especially any "cold" liquids. The water she did give him, however, came from the nearby jui (irrigation ditch). Since the water flowed continuously, Bibi Khanom knew it was safe to drink.

The situation began to appear desperate to Gul Jan. He was convinced that Ahmad Shah would die unless he received help soon. But what could he do? Finally Gul Jan made a decision. He would take Ahmad Shah directly to Kabul and find one of the big gleaming new hospitals there. If anyone could help Ahmad Shah, a doctor in Kabul should be able to.

Postscript: Ahmad Shah died shortly after reaching Kabul. The doctor said it was pneumonia and that Gul Jan had come too late.

A. Introduction

The Basic Health Centers of rural Afghanistan, even if increased in number and improved in quality, are incapable of providing easily accessible primary health care to the 85 percent of Afghanistan's population living in remote villages. The surveys conducted by the Ministry and the team in 1974–1976 demonstrated unequivocally that utilization of Basic Health Centers was to a very large extent by villagers living within a 10-kilometer radius. The question remained: What do we do about the majority of the population living more than 10 kilometers from a center?

These rural people, for whom the closest center is still too far, rely for their health care on a system of indigenous practitioners and traditional remedies. In the town bazaar, and less often in the villages, there are *hakimji* (traditional practitioners), *mullahs* (holy men), injectionists, barbers, *dais* (traditional midwives), *dokhandars* (shopkeepers), *atars* (vendors of herbal medicines), and pharmacists to provide a variety of services. Nonetheless, no Western-style curative care is available for the many common ailments that beset this rural population, and more than one-third of Afghan infants die before reaching 5 years of age.

Clearly there is a need for the development of new approaches to primary health care, approaches to complement the existing BHC system and extend the provision of care beyond its confines. During 1975 and 1976, the Ministry began to consider alternative programs in the context of (1) its technical and managerial capacity to sustain new approaches and (2) the external environment in which it operated.

The Ministry was aware that real constraints existed in its ability to plan and to staff whatever programs were likely to emerge. There was a hesitancy among senior officials to accept responsible roles in health planning because these were seen as high-risk positions that had significant potential for visible failure as well as conflict with other Ministry departments. Manpower-development problems remained another important deficiency in the Ministry's capacity to develop and sustain new programs. Furthermore, limitations of government funds made it clear that a primary requirement in health-system design was the minimization of direct government operating costs. For these reasons and others, the management team took an active role—and many of the risks—in the planning of an Alternative Health Delivery System (AHDS).

Feasibility considerations in the development of a new program involved a survey of current activities in rural areas. Several successful "vertical" health programs operated independently in Afghanistan: 900 malaria-surveillance agents took blood smears from villagers and provided some follow-up; mobile mass-immunization teams (originally smallpox vaccinators) had been very effective in serving remote areas; and rural water-supply programs also were administered with varying degrees of effectiveness. Other programs with impact in rural areas operated through the Ministry of Education, the Ministry of Agriculture, the Rural Development Department, and the Military. They offered potential for coordination with health initiatives, although the current administrative climate favored distinct and separate functioning.

In this setting, the Ministry arrived at several alternatives for consideration in extending primary health care beyond the BHC. These included the following:

Building more BHCs or subcenters. This alternative required a very high initial capital cost for constructing the centers as well as very high recurring costs for staffing, supplying, and maintaining the centers. A basic constraint was that the Ministry was not adequately staffing or supplying its existing health centers. Building more centers would only exacerbate the problem.

Training existing government health workers (especially malaria and smallpox workers) to deliver primary health care in villages. This option was seriously considered by the Ministry, but rejected because of the fear that these workers might neglect some of their critically important duties in immunization or malaria control. The Ministry recognized that once malaria or smallpox field workers could legally dispense drugs, nothing else in their new job descriptions would have much appeal.

Another approach considered by the Ministry involved *using village schools for an intense health-education and health-promotion campaign.* However, village schools were administered by the Ministry of Education, and interministerial cooperation has always been very difficult to achieve in Afghanistan. Also, any village-school program would not directly involve mothers and their children under 5—the most vulnerable groups and the highest priority for any village health program.

A fourth alternative was to *train already existing indigenous practitioners* at the village level.

A fifth and final major option that was considered by the Ministry was to have *villagers choose someone from among themselves* (not necessarily a traditional healer) *to be trained as a village health worker* [*VHW*].

Obviously, these alternatives were not mutually exclusive possibilities. All of them were explored, and within two years, the Ministry had developed the information necessary for planning Alternative Health Delivery

Systems (AHDS) using the fourth and fifth strategies. The limits of the BHC system were known; surveys had established what the rural health environment was like beyond the reach of current Ministry programs; the pitfalls in and potentially improvable aspects of central management systems were known; and financial constraints were understood. Table 3–1 summarizes the salient facts and implications underlying the AHDS strategies.

Recognizing the potential importance and uniqueness of the diverse settings—cultural, economic, and geoclimatic—encompassed by Afghanistan, the Ministry elected to test two approaches in different settings in a phased, sequential fashion. The *village health worker* approach was the first chosen, for three reasons: (1) there was demonstrated rural interest, and it promised to provide new local jobs for local people; (2) the Ministry realized that foreign donors (such as WHO, UNICEF, and USAID) were very interested in this kind of program and donor money was available; and (3) there was no existing model or tradition, and hence limited internal resistance could be expected. Indigenous practitioners, *dokhandars,* and pharmacists were all established images, good or bad, and therefore had both advocates and adversaries at a time when the Ministry was primarily interested in protecting these first steps from preformed opinion.

The VHW would be concerned chiefly with curative medicine, environmental health, immunization, and health education. To handle maternal and child care, it was decided to offer training to the traditional village *dais* (traditional midwives), who were already practitioners in their villages. This was the first time in Afghanistan that a category of traditional practitioners received official recognition from the government. The VHW and the *dai,* working ideally as a team, would together serve the basic health needs of the rural area.

The proposed AHDS were presented first to the Cabinet and then publicly as the first of a series of trials of different models. The program offered (1) an innovative combination of government resources for initial training and village self-support for continued operation, and (2) a flexible adaptive approach, acknowledging that different models might well be called for in diverse areas of the country. The Village Health Worker Program is discussed in section 3.B, the *Dai* Program in section 3.C.

B. The Village Health Worker Program
Steven L. Solter and *Peter N. Cross*

Introduction

The Ministry of Public Health first considered the idea of village health workers (VHWs) in the fall of 1973, when MSH arrived in the country.

Table 3–1

Facts to Be Considered in Alternative Health-Delivery-Systems Planning

Facts	Implications
1. Majority of the rural population lived beyond 6 to 10 km or 1 hour travel-time radius of BHC service.	BHCs could at best serve from one-quarter to one-third of the rural population.
2. The Ministry had limited ability to provide trained manpower.	Any new AHDS should not rely on highly trained personnel such as doctors, nurses, and nurse-midwives.
3. The Ministry did not have the financial capacity to provide free health services to the entire population.	No fixed government-operated facilities were likely beyond the BHC level for the indefinite future. The AHDS should be largely self-supporting.
4. The drug-supply logistics system could be improved slowly.	Basic drugs could be supplied to BHCs and to a slowly expanded AHDS.
5. Rural Afghans: Were very interested in health and pursued multiple avenues of care. Were interested in having local residents trained as health agents. Already invest a lot of their own resources seeking health care. Desired local access to modern medicines more than physicians or hospitals.	Rural interest in supporting local health agents trained by the Ministry would be sustained. Rural Afghans would be willing to transfer some of their current health expenditures to pay for services of new local health agents and for drugs provided by them.

Early discussions between high-level MOPH officials, including the Minister, and management team advisors suggested that the only way Afghanistan could provide accessible primary health care to the majority of its population (living in 23,000 villages, many of them very remote) was by training large numbers of VHWs. But this was not an idea easily acceptable to senior Ministry staff.

Most high-level Ministry officials at that time were physicians who had graduated from an Afghan medical school and who had had relatively little experience either outside the country or, being urban elite, with village health problems within Afghanistan. The central idea of the VHW—that villagers choose someone from their village with minimal education to be trained in a brief course in a nearby BHC and return to the village to treat common medical problems and provide basic health education—was a concept foreign to Afghan doctors and Ministry officials and was not immediately welcome. Gradually, as the Chinese "barefoot doctor" became better known, as Afghan Ministry officials were invited to conferences on village health workers (such as the one held in Shiraz, Iran, in 1975), and as WHO's position supporting primary health care became clear, the atmosphere in Kabul grew more supportive of the idea. Although some misgivings and grave doubts persisted, the MOPH fully realized by early 1976 that the major international donors (such as AID, WHO, and UNICEF) were firmly committed to extending health care to villagers through the use of VHWs.

Thus, in the spring of 1976, the Ministry and AID decided to support several "experiments" in creating Alternative Health Delivery Systems (AHDS) in the MOPH. A three-province survey conducted in Baghlan, Ghazni, and Helmand provinces between August and October 1976 documented the degree of interest, as well as the specific suggestions, of 723 randomly selected adult villagers living in seventeen different villages throughout the three provinces. Of the villagers interviewed, 90 percent felt that a VHW program was feasible for their own village. The majority of villagers interviewed believed that villagers themselves should select their own VHWs. The majority of respondents also felt that VHWs should be literate and could be either male or female.

Although the results of this large survey did not seem to particularly interest most MOPH officials, the fact that the great majority of villagers supported the idea of VHWs was useful information for those few individuals in the Ministry who were interested in the program. The data provided a means to counter objections to the VHW concept that were frequently raised, for example, that "the villagers will never accept such a poorly trained, low-level health worker." Rather than providing only "objective" information to help decision makers arrive at rational decisions, surveys in Afghanistan supported various factions in the political decisions they made. This survey was thus used as a post facto means of justification for the new VHW concept.

Once the MOPH was convinced that a VHW Program should begin, it sought and obtained approval from the Afghan cabinet in April of 1977. Consent was given for a program to train 1,500 VHWs throughout the country by 1982. These 1,500 VHWs would provide basic coverage for only about 10 percent of the rural population. Funds for training, per diem, supplies, and each VHW's initial stock of drugs would come from UNICEF; technical assistance was provided by AID through its contract with MSH.

Cabinet approval was not as difficult for the Minister to obtain as the team feared. The MOPH was considered a "technical" Ministry, capable of making "technical decisions" on its own. Furthermore, since the VHW program was to take place almost entirely in villages and did not conflict with the interests of other Ministries, it was politically acceptable and therefore passed without significant opposition.

So the VHW program was underway. The first group of eleven VHWs completed training in May of 1977; between that time and January of 1979 (when the program ended), a total of 137 VHWs were trained. The management team concentrated its efforts toward solving the operational problems of the expanding program in an attempt to ensure its survival. The new pro-Soviet government that took power in Kabul in April of 1978 decided to eliminate the VHW program for political rather than technical reasons. New advisors urged the Ministry to stop training workers similar to the Chinese "barefoot doctors." They argued that health workers similar to the Soviet *feldshers* should be trained instead. Despite the fact that *feldshers* were inappropriate for providing health care to Afghan villagers (since they came from the city, were not chosen by the villagers, and were based in fixed health facilities located at a great distance from many villages), the MOPH decided to accept the Soviet advice.

In September of 1978, there was an International Conference on Primary Health Care (sponsored by WHO and UNICEF) held in Alma Ata, U.S.S.R. The leader of the Afghan delegation was the Deputy Minister of Health, an inexperienced 26-year-old nephew of the then Foreign Minister, and later President Hafizullah Amin. It is interesting to note that prior to the Alma Ata meeting, the Deputy Health Minister was a strong public supporter of VHWs. When he returned from the meeting, he was determined to destroy the program, even at the risk of alienating international donors. It appears that while at Alma Ata, the Deputy Minister was persuaded to abandon a program that smacked of Chinese origins.

Such was the determination of the new Afghan government's health officials and their Soviet advisors that MSH, USAID, UNICEF, and WHO were unable to save the VHW program. Discussions within the MOPH of increasing the number of trained VHWs from 1,500 to 15,000 were curtailed and the possibility of Afghanistan being one of the first developing countries to provide accessible primary care to the majority of its population had to be abandoned for the forseeable future.

This, then, is the short history of the team involvement in the training of village health workers. A major evaluative effort had been scheduled for 1979 which would have documented the extent to which Afghan VHWs were able to influence villagers' health knowledge and health practices. This would have been achieved by a repeat survey planned to follow-up the baseline survey conducted in Ghazni province in 1977. In the baseline survey, the health knowledge and health practices of villagers living in areas where there would soon be a VHW were compared with those in areas where there would be no VHWs. Thus a follow-up survey could observe whether VHWs themselves were responsible for any improvements in health knowledge and health practices among their fellow villagers. In addition, much more information would have become available on drug flow and VHW usage. Following a fuller explanation of the VHW program, existing data concerning VHW performance, will be analyzed.

VHW Program Development: Defining the VHW Role

Once the political decision had been made to go ahead with a VHW Program, the team suggested that interested MOPH officials meet on a regular basis in order to decide who these workers should be and what they should be trained to do. Beginning in October of 1976, a series of informal "luncheon" meetings was held in which specific aspects (such as recruitment and selection, training, supervision, supply, continuing education, and evaluation) were discussed. In retrospect, a number of hotly debated and important decisions were made at these meetings that had a profound influence over the future of the project. Each decision was ultimately made by consensus, so that every individual attending the meetings had to make a number of compromises, but MOPH officials were responsible for all final decisions.

How Would the VHWs Be Chosen? It had already been decided that VHWs would be selected by their villages, but there remained several options as to guidelines for selection. The MOPH could insist that all VHWs chosen by villagers *must* be already practicing traditional healers. This would have two major advantages. If only indigenous practitioners could become VHWs, then Afghan doctors would be less likely to oppose them, because their training would merely enable them to do better that which they have already been doing anyway. The second advantage would be the fact that villagers were already visiting them for health reasons, and their upgraded status would simply help them be more effective in changing health habits. There would also be disadvantages in requiring VHWs to be former traditional healers. For one thing, it would greatly limit the freedom of choice of villagers. In addition, traditional healers could be reluctant in many ways to make fundamental changes in their practices: a barber who has made his living by doing minor surgery for 30 years may not readily adjust to a different philosophy of health care.

The second option was to allow the villages complete freedom to choose anyone they wanted to be their VHW. This, of course, could result in close relatives of village leaders being chosen. However, this would allow villagers to take a more active role in making those decisions which affected their lives.

The third alternative was to strongly suggest to villagers that a traditional healer be chosen as their VHW, but not make it compulsory. Also considered a strong contender for the VHW role was the local village shopkeeper, or *dokhandar*. Unlike many government-supplied institutions, the private *dokhans* (shops) were nearly always stocked with the things people wanted to buy. The *dokhandars* knew how to maintain their supplies, were centrally located, were open long hours, and could be trained to give health advice and sell basic drugs for common conditions.

The MOPH finally decided to leave the ultimate VHW choice completely up to the villagers. Whether they chose a traditional healer, a *dokhandar,* or anyone else was their decision.

Setting Minimum Qualifications: Several issues had to be clarified before rational minimum qualifications for VHWs could be determined. First of all, if the villagers, or the "village committee" elected by them, were responsible for selecting their VHW, than any a priori minimum qualifications that might be set by the MOPH would interfere with the villagers' freedom to choose. However, if each village chose whomever it wanted without paying attention to minimum standards or criteria, was there then a risk that the *Khan*'s feeble-minded son might be chosen? Furthermore, without a requirement for literacy, for example, each VHW class might consist of both literates and illiterates, greatly complicating the training process.

This fundamental dilemma was resolved by the MOPH by providing guidelines for the "Village Committee," but respecting the final decision of the village even if some of the guidelines were violated. The major guidelines were that the VHW should be

Functionally literate;

Older than 18 years;

If male, finished with his military obligations;

Able to spend at least 4 hours per day as a VHW;

Accepted by all major factions in the village;

Dedicated to serving his fellow villagers;

Intelligent and honest;

Respected by his fellow villagers.

Another crucial issue concerned the sex of the VHW. Ministry officials concerned with establishing a VHW program recognized the fact that a female health worker was more likely to influence village child-care and child-feeding practices (as well as contraceptive behavior) than would a male health worker. The difficulty lay in the fact the female VHWs might not be allowed to leave their villages for training, were not likely to be literate, and being illiterate, would not be good candidates for providing basic drugs (since Afghan physicians were likely to violently oppose illiterate village females distributing any kind of drug whatsoever). The MOPH at first considered allowing only literate female VHWs to have drugs, but there were so few literate village women available as VHWs that this idea was soon abandoned in practice. Instead, the Ministry decided to train men as VHWs in the areas of basic curative care, environmental sanitation, and personal hygiene and to simultaneously train traditional village midwives (*dais*, who were largely illiterate) in the areas of maternal/child health (MCH) and family planning. In this way, a basic team consisting of a VHW and a *dai* could provide the essential primary health-care services at the village level, easily accessible to the great majority of the population.

Skills and Competence: It was important to define the context in which the VHW would function and to *determine the skills and competencies he or she should possess*. Since the major health problems of the village were considered to be preventable morbidity and mortality in children under 5 as well as uncontrolled fertility, blamed partly on certain long-standing health habits, it was felt that a trained VHW could be most effective by trying to encourage changes in these habits. Some of the most important practices and beliefs that the Ministry felt were detrimental to village health are listed below:

Infants were usually fed only breast milk until 24 months of age, with little supplementation.

Infants and young children with diarrhea were not rehydrated by their parents.

Sick children were usually given inadequate fluids and not fed properly because of traditional beliefs concerning diet and disease.

Any flowing water was considered safe for drinking.

Most villagers did not wash hands with soap and water prior to preparing food, before eating, or after defecating.

Flies and feces were ubiquitous and constantly contaminating food and water.

Based on these observations, it was clear that the VHW curriculum would have to stress practical approaches to health education, nutrition, personal hygiene, and environmental health. In addition, VHWs would have to be able to provide effective contraceptives (for the first time in any Afghan government-supported program) as well as basic drugs for common complaints. Another essential would be to distinguish those patients whom the VHW could treat in the village from those patients needing referral to the BHC. Underlying all was the importance of the VHW serving as a model by practicing those health habits which he or she was telling others to practice.

The Length of Initial VHW Training: Training was fixed at 3 weeks (6 hours per day and 6 days per week), but only after substantial debate among MOPH officials. Several officials contended that if the majority of Afghanistan's 23,000 villages were to have a VHW within a reasonable period of time, the length of training would have to be kept to a minimum. They further argued that a longer training period would be too costly in terms of training personnel and per diems, and that a 2- or 3-week period was long enough for the basic, essential skills needed to substantially reduce preventable child mortality in the village. Further training could be given in the form of short, intensive continuing-education courses.

Others, however, suggested that in order to persuade Afghan doctors that VHWs possessed minimal skills, a longer period of training was essential. They felt that a villager who had had a limited education (4 years, for example) and who had completed his education in a village school 10 years before would need a certain minimum length of time to become adjusted to completely alien ways of thought. It also was pointed out that many VHWs would probably have been indigenous practitioners in their villages and that it takes time to train such workers to be able to effectively combine traditional and modern medicine. The final decision, favoring the short course, was based primarily on the argument of the overwhelming numbers to be trained and the very limited resources with which to accomplish such an enormous task.

Drug Dispensing: Whether VHWs Would Dispense Drugs: This also generated a great deal of controversy. Once again, a major area of disagreement was the potential impact of this decision on the opinion of Afghan physicians. Some MOPH officials felt that a few key drugs (such as oral penicillin or a glucose electrolyte mix for diarrhea and dehydration) could be lifesaving in remote villages where bacterial pneumonia and dehydration were leading causes of death in children under 5 years of age. They argued that without such essential drugs, the likelihood of the VHW having a significant impact on child mortality was minimal. In addition, villagers were mostly interested in drugs for the relief of illness; a VHW whose armamentarium was limited to advice on how to live in a healthy manner would be ignored or even possibly shunned. The MOPH officials suggested that VHWs who could provide basic curative care for common conditions would be much more influential in changing harmful health habits than would a VHW who was not able to treat those who came to him or her.

An opposing group within the Ministry argued that if the VHWs were allowed to dispense drugs, this would be so threatening to the Afghan doctors (since the self-image of Afghan doctors is largely that of someone who prescribes drugs) that the program would be doomed. In addition, all drugs can cause side effects and complications; if a villager were treated by a

VHW and the treatment were followed by some untoward reaction, the villager would blame the VHW and the program could become discredited. Furthermore, drugs must be continuously resupplied. If the MOPH has difficulty supplying 120 BHCs with drugs, how would it ever be able to supply 15,000 VHWs on a continuous basis? It was stated that it would be better for a VHW to have no drugs than to have drugs initially only to run out of them at a later date. A final argument of this faction was that to allow VHWs to prescribe drugs would mean that, in effect, the VHWs would do very little other than curative care, since the villagers would be far more interested in drugs than in health education and there would be almost no incentive for the VHW to provide any preventive services.

Consensus was finally reached to allow the VHWs to prescribe drugs, but whether they should give injections was an emotion-laden issue. It was recognized that villagers generally prefer injections to tablets, capsules, or syrups (the more painful the injection the better—if it hurts, it must be good), and if the VHW were to have any status or respect in the village, it was essential that he or she be able to give injections. It also was recognized that nearly every village has an untrained injectionist whose technique is likely to be decidedly unsterile; if the VHWs did not give injections, then villagers would surely seek that service from the local injectionists. It was thus decided that VHWs should be taught how to give injections using sterile technique, although they should not be provided any injectable drugs by the MOPH. Only oral drugs would be provided to the VHWs.

Further debate led to the following list of drugs that VHWs could prescribe. All were to be prepackaged in course-of-treatment dosage packages.

Tetracycline eye ointment (to be used topically for conjunctivitis and for the early stages of trachoma);

Aspirin;

Penicillin V (oral, to be given only when the patient had cough and a body temperature greater than 38°C);

Oral contraceptives;

Piperazine (for roundworm infections, which are extremely prevalent in Afghan villages);

Ferrous sulfate with folate (iron, for anemia, which is particularly common in adult Afghan women);

Multivitamins with iron (including vitamin A for xerophthalmia);

Oral rehydration salts (a glucose-electrolyte solution for diarrhea and dehydration. Some VHWs also were provided simple antacids and sulfadimidine).

These particular drugs were chosen because each of them was considered effective against conditions or problems that were an important cause of morbidity and/or mortality in the village and because each (with the exception of oral contraceptives) was quite safe, even when given in very large dosages. Even if a particularly avaricious VHW prescribed every different drug packet every day to everyone in his village, the resulting harm should be minimal.

The VHWs were unhappy with the fact that they did not receive an antidiarrheal drug. The glucose-electrolyte packets were for replacing vital fluids and salts lost from the body during an episode of diarrhea, but they could not *stop* the diarrhea. Afghan physicians prescribe antidiarrheals to young children with diarrhea (the favorite drug is Sulfaguanidine), and fluid and salt replacement are rarely emphasized to the parent. Consequently, a large number of Afghan children die from dehydration, even after being seen by a physician. Had the VHWs been able to dispense Sulfaguanidine routinely, in addition to the glucose-electrolyte packet, it is likely that they would have dispensed only the Sulfaguanidine (since that was the drug that the villagers were used to), and dehydration in children would have gone uncorrected. Similar discussions and arguments took place with regard to all the VHW drugs. Those selected for inclusion in the VHW armamentarium were felt to be appropriate both at the start of the program and after 18 months of field experience.

Program Financing: The VHW was not salaried by the Afghan government, but would be allowed to sell prepackaged drugs at a small profit. There was very little disagreement on this issue. MOPH officials shared the view that the government was not prepared to pay VHW salaries from its meager budget and recognized that international donors are usually very reluctant to pay salaries except as a temporary measure. All agreed that the VHW should be compensated in some fashion for his or her work, but felt that this support should come from the villages.

The rural health surveys had revealed a startling fact, that the mean annual personal-health expenditure in rural Afghanistan is seven times the government expenditure. This meant that 87.5 percent of all money spent on health care in Afghanistan comes out of the pockets of impoverished villagers, representing 7.4 percent of the annual household income of the average Afghan family. Closer examination of this household health expenditure disclosed the importance of drugs to the Afghan: he spends 37 percent of his health "dollar" on pharmacy drugs and additional money on traditional herbs and medicines. The willing expenditure for drugs suggested a means of support for the new village-based health program.

Since villagers were interested in having a VHW, and since they were willing to pay for drugs, the Ministry decided that VHWs could sell their drugs at a small profit (2 Afghani or 5 cents per packet). A village could supplement this income—by allowing the VHW to charge on a fee-for-service basis or by asking each household to contribute a certain amount in Afhanis per month—but this was to be decided by each community for itself. It also was generally agreed that each VHW should have some other job or means of support, that being a VHW should not be a full-time job.

The Process of VHW Selection

Start-up of the VHW Program required interaction and cooperation between Afghan villages and the central government, since, by design, village health workers were to be chosen by their villages and trained nearby at BHCs by government (donor-supported) teams. Traditionally, however, the government in Kabul has been viewed with suspicion by many villagers, and especially by nomads. The fierce independent spirit of Pathan (pushtun) tribes is legendary and continues to this day. Thus a new government program must recognize this ingrained suspicion and work to overcome it, eliciting the support of villagers as a precondition for any degree of success.

Villagers are first and foremost pragmatists. If a program meets a basic unmet need, and if there is no hint of exploitation, they will support it. Centuries of experience have taught them to be wary; and if a clear benefit is perceived, the support of villagers can reach a high level, as demonstrated in both the smallpox-eradication and the malaria-control programs.

With this in mind, the VHW Program undertook to visit villages located far (at least 10 kilometers) from the nearest BHC in order to determine if there was any interest in the program. Consistent with the Three-Province Survey results (in which villagers expressed great interest in the idea), the VHW recruitment teams received an enthusiastic response in nearly every village they visited. Having one of their own people trained in health care and equipped with basic drugs fulfilled a universal need. Many villagers were at first suspicious, but the desire to have their own trained health worker was so strong that most hesitations were short-lived.

An important lesson that can be drawn from the involvement of the Afghan government in conservative, traditional village communities has been the importance of working through the existing power structure. Afghan villages are not democratic in the Western sense and never have been. Decisions are made by consensus, with village elders and powerful landlords having disproportionate influence over the outcome. If these village leaders are bypassed by trying to have all villagers express their opinions, in a one-man, one-vote kind of election, confusion and program failure inevitably result. The Afghan village may someday be transformed, but it will not happen as a byproduct of a government health program.

Thus, although community participation should remain a goal to be sought after, program planners cannot afford to be naive about village realities.

Village Committees: A fundamental assumption of the VHW Program was that success depended on active community participation in all phases of the program. The key feature of VHW recruitment was the creation of "village committees." These village committees, consisting of three to five men chosen by the villagers themselves, had the responsibility of selecting the VHW for their village, supporting him in his work (including ensuring that he had an adequate "clinic" room), and making sure that he performed honestly and competently.

A VHW recruitment team (usually consisting of two sanitarians and a driver) spent an average of 2 weeks recruiting fifteen to twenty VHWs in a single *woleswali* (or district), visiting villages located at least 10 kilometers from the BHC of the *woleswali.* The principal task of the recruitment team was to help set up functioning village committees. The experience of recruiting eighty-three VHWs in six different *woleswalis* can be summarized as follows. In the majority of villages, the first person consulted by the recruitment team was the most important man in the village (variously known as the *malek, arbab, carriodar,* or *khan*). This man then called together the other important village elders (known as *risch safid,* or "white beards"). Together they decided who would be members of the village committee (*kilay jirga*). Usually the same men who informally made decisions anyway for the village were the ones selected.

Although the VHW recruitment teams made every effort to convince the village committees to take their new responsibility seriously, this in fact rarely turned out to be the case. The village committee members were invariably polite and agreed to anything that the recruitment teams suggested. However, when the village was subsequently visited by the VHW supervisor (after the VHW had begun working in the village), the village committee in most cases had not done what it had promised to do. For example, in many villages the village committee members had promised to make available a room for the VHW to use as his clinic. When these villages had been visited months later by a VHW supervisor, the promised clinic rooms had generally not been provided. When asked the reason why, the village committee members usually shrugged and promised once again that they would do it. It seems clear that although the village committees were usually well-meaning and supportive (even enthusiastic) about their VHWs, they were rarely willing to take concrete steps that required time and money because of a belief that if they did not do it, perhaps the government would.

At the onset of the VHW Program, one of the chief concerns of the recruitment teams was that many Afghan villages would be faction-ridden and that there would be major disagreements between the factions over the choice of a VHW and over how he should be supervised. However, only one village is known to have suffered from factional problems regarding their VHW (in Jaji Maidan, Paktia Province). If factions were a major problem in other villages, this was not observed by either recruitment or supervisory teams.

Profile of VHWs Trained: Most of the VHWs selected by the village committees can be divided into three groups. One group consisted of young, literate, underemployed men who were sons or nephews of members of the village committee. A typical member of this group might be a 24-year-old son of a prominent *malek*. The *malek* had three older sons to work his land, but there was not enough land to support his youngest son as well. This youngest son was then selected to be a VHW, thereby gaining some prestige and a small income for this part-time job. The second group of VHWs included *mullahs* and shopkeepers, who were usually literate and respected in the village. The third group consisted of literate men who had been indigenous practitioners of some sort, most often as injectionists, herbalists, or bone-setters. Most of the VHWs selected were genuinely interested in the job of VHW.

Overall, of the 137 VHWs trained during the life of the project, the typical worker was male (only six were female) and about 34 years old. (The youngest was a 15-year-old nomad, while the oldest was a 57-year-old *mullah*.) He was literate (although minimally) and had probably attended school for about four years. (Many elder VHWs had acquired literacy through informal teachings of the local *mullah*, although one elderly VHW was a retired military officer who had a degree from a military college.) Eighty persent of the VHWs were married, and 91 percent had completed their military obligation. As table 3–2 shows, most VHWs were farmers.

As the Program Evolved: Observations, Problems, and Constraints

Training of VHWs: The fundamental principle underlying the training of VHWs was that a short, practical training course (utilizing clear-cut teaching objectives) could transmit simple skills which, when applied under village conditions, could be effective in lowering morbidity and mortality rates, particularly among children under five and among pregnant and lactating women.

The Afghan VHW training course lasted 3 weeks and was conducted at the Basic Health Center in the *woleswali* where the VHW villages were located. The VHWs stayed at the BHC or at the homes of relatives nearby, since their villages were often 20 or 30 kilometers away from the BHC. The

Table 3–2
Main Occupations of Village Health Workers

Occupation	Number of VHWs	Percentage of VHWs
Farmers	79	58
Shopkeepers/itinerant traders	18	13
Mullahs	14	10
Housewives	6	4
Unemployed	6	4
Laborers	6	4
Nomad/shepherd	3	2
Traditional-medicine practitioners	1	1
Others (including one unknown)	4	3
Total	137	99

course was run by a VHW training team consisting of two sanitarians (from Kabul) trained in teaching methods and in the use of the VHW curriculum. The class size ranged from approximately ten to twenty students, with nearly all VHWs being literate males.

Since the Afghan VHW Program never was expanded, the small Kabul-based staff was able to conduct all the training courses themselves. Had there been a major expansion, however, new trainers would have learned how to train VHWs by joining trainers already on the job, with periodic in-service training to upgrade their skills, particularly in practical teaching methods that deemphasize the use of lectures.

Response of the VHWs to Training Efforts: The VHWs were extremely eager to learn and seized the opportunity with great enthusiasm. Many had read all 150 pages of their textual material by the second or third day of the 3-week training program. By the end of the program, many VHW trainees had nearly memorized much of the material through continual rereading. They frequently kept trainers after class to discuss their village's health problems. It would be hard to imagine a more enthusiastic group of students.

There was, however, a difference between the younger and older trainees in their ability to integrate what they were taught and to use their new knowledge in their village work. Supervisory visits after training to older VHWs (particularly *mullahs* and shopkeepers and those who had been injectionists or indigenous practitioners) revealed that they had difficulty changing some of their health practices. Younger VHWs, however, while not having health beliefs or practices of long standing that were resistant to change, were not as well respected by their fellow villagers as were their older colleagues. Thus VHW recruitment and training faced a dilemma. If younger VHWs were trained, they were much more likely than older VHWs to follow the principles and behaviors they had been taught, but their health-education advice was not as likely to be followed. Since the villagers themselves made the final selection of VHWs, the VHW training teams had to do the best job they could with whomever the villagers chose.

Pretests and Posttests: Pretests and posttests were considered essential to measure changes in knowledge that had taken place during VHW training. Each trainee took a twenty-question oral pretest prior to the start of his training and an oral posttest consisting of the same twenty questions after the 3-week training program. Both pretest and posttest scores are available for seventy-one VHWs. The average score on the pretest was 41.3 out of a possible 100. Scores ranged from 7 up to 68. After training, the scores improved to an average of 83.9, with a range of 71 to 95. On the basis of these scores, all VHWs were awarded official certificates indicating their satisfactory completion of training.

Follow-up "post-posttests" were given at the time of the first continuing-education course. These were again the same questions, administered 3 or more months after completion of initial training, and they were important as a means of determining whether the skills originally taught were still being practiced. The average score on these post-posttests was 86.6, suggesting that the VHWs retained their learning well. Improvement over posttest scores may have been due to familiarity with the test or the result of VHWs studying their reference books.

Test results demonstrated consistently high levels of performance by VHWs both young and old, thus pointing unreservedly to the ability of villagers to master the knowledge and skills required of a VHW. Similar evidence of their learning capacity was provided by eight VHW trainees who were given a special 3-day continuing-education course in immunization. The average pretest score was 21. Posttest scores averaged 85, a 300 percent improvement.

Experience with VHWs in training indicates that oral examinations given individually are preferable to written tests, although they take more time. The questions should test those practical skills which are the most important for the functions the VHW is to fulfill—ultimately reducing morbidity and mortality in the village. Results of the tests could be additionally useful in pointing out which parts of the curriculum are not being effectively taught and in thus evaluating the effectiveness of individual trainers.

Curriculum and Training Skills: Fundamental to successful VHW training was the development of a simple, appropriate training curriculum designed to train literate villagers. A set of three manuals were developed (in Dari and Pashto) to assist the VHW in learning basic skills and in performing necessary curative and preventive tasks in the village. By using the manuals, the VHW could "look up" anything he was unable to remember.

For example, if a VHW saw a patient with an eye complaint, he could look up eye problems in either his Reference Manual or his Field Manual. The Reference Manual discussed, in a clear and simple way, what kinds of eye problems were common in the village and what could be done about them. The Field Manual, in a more specific and concrete way, stated when an eye patient should be referred to the BHC doctor and when such a patient could be treated by the VHW in the village. It also listed several key points necessary for the prevention of eye diseases in villages that the VHW should explain to the patient. In addition, it listed exactly what should be done about treating eye problems.

The VHW curriculum initially emphasized the training of VHWs to perform those skills listed in the manuals. The curriculum was divided into the following areas: maternal and child health (and family planning), environmental sanitation, personal hygiene, nutrition, introduction to the human body and germ theory of disease, first aid, curative medical care, immunization, and organization of the VHW's job. Principles and techniques of health education and of working with community leaders (such as the village committee) were stressed throughout the 3-week course.

Practical work was to be given the highest priority, but became the most serious problem faced by the training teams. The plan was that VHWs would spend a considerable portion of their training time actually *doing* the things they would do on their own in the village, such as providing first aid, rehydrating children with diarrhea, teaching villagers about the importance of clean drinking water, and so forth, but since the 3-week courses were conducted at BHCs, the trainers had to depend on patients at the BHC for all curative and first-aid teaching. Some BHCs had very few patients for a variety of reasons. If, during the 3-week course, no patients with burns or fractures came to the BHC, the VHW trainers were forced to teach the diagnosis and treatment of these conditions by lecture or demonstration using normal subjects. The training teams found, however, that by being imaginative with those patients who did come to the BHC, they could provide the VHWs with adequate practical training.

Nonetheless, some VHW trainers were not very imaginative in making the training practical. As products themselves of the Afghan educational system, which utilizes lectures almost exclusively as a means of transmitting information and skills, they often preferred to lecture rather than to have the students actually practice those tasks which they would have to perform

when they returned to their villages. Despite on-the-job training to emphasize the "practical," they persisted in giving lectures. This problem contributed to a decision to revise the VHW curriculum to help improve the quality
of teaching practical skills to VHWs. The revised curriculum was completed
and first field-tested in October of 1978. It was determined to be an
improvement, but was short-lived because the VHW Program came to an
end a few months later.

Summary of 18 Months of Experience with the Afghan VHW Curriculum:
For a curriculum to be effective, it must be very specific and detailed; each
point should be made clearly and distinctly, and examples of how that
teaching point can be taught should be made explicit for the trainers. All
trainers must themselves be trained in using the curriculum, preferably by
both classroom teaching and on-the-job training. In order to use the VHW
curriculum most effectively, the training teams, when in the field, must be
able to purchase certain items (like locally available weaning foods) which
are essential for teaching. The trainers must periodically have "refresher
courses" themselves, so that their interest in the curriculum remains active
and alive. The curriculum must be revised reasonably often, with the trainers providing the most important input. And finally, audiovisual and other
teaching aids should be integrated with the curriculum in order to have the
greatest possible impact.

Support of VHWs through Supervision and Supply: The support of
VHWs—through supervision and supply—proved to be far more difficult
to maintain than was the training component. While a great deal of time
and energy was spent in developing manuals, teaching aids, and curricula,
less time and energy were devoted to the development of an effective supervisory system, and supervision of VHWs never reached a level that was
satisfactory to the Ministry.

The original design required the BHC sanitarian (who had assisted the
Kabul-based VHW training team) to visit each VHW in his *woleswali* once
per month. A detailed "supervisory checklist" was developed so that the
sanitarian knew exactly what he was supposed to do once he got to the
VHW village. Also, each checklist was keyed to a 100-point scale, so that
each VHW's performance could be evaluated monthly and compared with
his performance during previous months. However, the BHC sanitarians in
most cases failed to make their monthly supervisory visits.

The main reason the BHC sanitarians did not visit their VHWs was that
they lacked adequate incentive. The VHW, *dai,* and BHC training teams all
received substantial per diems (by Afghan standards) when they went to the
field. The BHC sanitarian, however, was never allowed by the MOPH to
receive more than the standard per diem; this was not easy to collect because

the MOPH required signatures as proof of travel and also stipulated that the trip must involve a certain minimum number of kilometers. Road conditions to most VHW villages were very poor, and adequate transportation for the sanitarian was often unavailable. All these factors combined, and the result was that VHW supervisory visits rarely took place. For a BHC sanitarian to have made frequent supervisory visits to VHWs required a level of commitment and dedication not often found in the MOPH or, for that matter, in any other health system. The "lesson" appears abundantly clear: unless there is adequate incentive (financial or otherwise, but usually financial), government-employed rural health workers are unlikely to suffer the difficult conditions involved in frequent field visits. When one considers their low pay (less than $60 per month), this should not be surprising. Only a political system that is able to generate a great deal of ideological zeal can expect its low-paid rural health workers to undergo great hardship with their only incentive being "to serve the people."

In addition to supervision, supply is the critical support need. Unlike the *dais,* who did not need to be resupplied (since they dispensed no drugs), the VHWs needed a continuous "pipeline" to keep them supplied with drugs and first-aid items, especially during the winter months when travel to Kabul or even to the BHC was very difficult. Each VHW was initially provided with approximately a 3-months supply of prepackaged drugs and a 1-year supply of first-aid materials. In addition, each VHW was given a metal storage cabinet with sixteen small drawers (so that each kind of drug or first-aid supply could be kept in a separate drawer). The VHWs were told that if they quit or were fired, they would have to return the cabinet and all drugs and supplies to the Ministry. After selling their initial stocks of drugs, the VHWs went to the nearest BHC to purchase additional packets of drugs.

Problems in Finding an Appropriate Financing Mechanism. After the Ministry decided to permit the workers to sell prepackaged drugs for a small profit (5 cents per packet) as well as to allow the village committees to decide on any other means of financial support for the VHW, it remained to be seen how this arrangement would work out in practice. Based on one and a half years of experience involving a total of about 130 VHWs, the following observations can be made.

None of the village committees were able to organize any system for financially supporting the VHWs. All the village committees were informed by VHW recruitment teams that they could allow the VHWs to charge a fee for service in addition to charging for drugs. The village committees also were told that they could require each household to pay a few Afghanis per month to supplement the VHW's income (as a kind of prepaid insurance scheme). When the village committees were visited at a later date and asked why they did not take these steps, the most frequent answer was that they were waiting for the VHW to receive a government salary. Despite repeated denials that this would, in fact, take place, most village committees rationalized their lack of financial support by insisting that a government salary was absolutely necessary.

The profit from the sale of prepackaged drugs, in itself, did not provide the VHWs with sufficient income to support a family. The average VHW sold no more than 100 packets per month (giving him a $5 monthly profit). Most VHWs, in addition, charged a small fee for giving injections and occasionally charged for providing first aid. Unless the VHW was able to earn substantially more money than this from some other job at the same time (such as farming or being a *mullah* or shopkeeper), he would have to quit being a VHW. What generally happened was that the men chosen to be VHWs either had no other job (and had to be subsidized anyway by their relatives) or were relatively affluent, as farmer, *mullah,* or shopkeeper, and could spare the time to be a VHW in order to gain the status and prestige associated with the job. The complaint about receiving no salary was a persistent one, however, affecting VHWs and village committee members alike. At the time the decision was made by the MOPH to end the VHW Program, a plan was under consideration in the MOPH to provide minimal monthly salaries to the VHWs. Had that plan gone into effect, assuming a salary of 1,000 Afghanis per month ($25) per VHW, the recurring government costs would have been approximately $4,500,000 per year for 15,000 VHWs (enough to provide 1:500 coverage), probably a prohibitive figure.

The MOPH on several occasions considered increasing the profit per packet allowed to the VHW. However, when the VHWs in Jaghori (Ghazni Province, in the Hazarajat) were asked if they favored an increased profit, they said no. The Jaghori VHWs at that time (in December of 1977) had already been working as VHWs for a number of months and understood their financial situation quite well. They felt that some villagers in that very poor area could barely afford the medicine they were selling (despite the fact that the drugs they sold, supplied by UNICEF, cost the villagers far less than the same drugs bought at a pharmacy). To raise the price per packet in order to give more profit to the VHWs would cause hardship. Also, such a rise in price would harm the very positive image the VHWs had acquired in their villages. It is possible that the Jaghori VHWs might have reconsidered their decision at a later date, but they never had the opportunity. When the new government took power in April of 1978, it made the promise that health services would be free. Although they allowed the VHWs to continue selling drugs for a number of months, Ministry officials were reluctant to ask the new Minister for increased profits for the VHWs; greater profits would be counter to the new regime's professed ideology.

Despite the frequently expressed fears of MOPH officials and others that the VHWs would cheat by either charging higher than allowed rates for their drug packets or else selling their UNICEF drugs to pharmacies at a big profit, there is no evidence to suggest that either was a common practice. Pharmacies sold the same drugs at prices 100 to 400 percent higher than what the VHWs were charging (and the pharmacies were usually located many kilometers from the VHWs' villages). This situation is ideal for a black market to be established. It is certainly possible that had thousands of VHWs been trained (instead of only 137), such a black market would have sprung up and the VHWs would have sold their UNICEF drugs to pharmacies. But as it happened, the great preponderance of UNICEF drugs were sold to villagers at the established rates. One reason for this may have been the fact that all the drug packets had labels which clearly showed what price of each was supposed to be. Also, the village committee had an interest in maintaining the correct price, since they benefited from the cheap prices along with everyone else. Finally, because the VHW Program was not allowed to expand as originally planned, there were always few enough VHWs so that selling drugs to pharmacies could be fairly easily noticed and reported. The prices of VHW drugs, therefore, appeared to be kept under control by a number of informal but effective mechanisms.

Curative Care Provided by VHWs: Village health workers kept a register book for all patients who came to them for curative services. Of 2,497 sequential patients seen by a sample of nine VHWs, the VHWs had recorded the problems of all but 109. Table 3-3 shows the relative frequency of all recorded problems. These results correspond quite closely to what had been anticipated on the basis of a report entitled "A Health Survey of Three Provinces of Afghanistan," published in November of 1977, as shown in table 3-4.

The discrepancies apparent in table 3-4 may have a reasonable explanation. Of the 2,497 patient visits analyzed, only 11 percent occurred during the period from December 21 to April 21. (This is explained largely by the uneven distribution of man-months of VHW service represented by the data being discussed. Of the sample's sixty-six man-months of VHW service, only ten and a half (16 percent) occurred between December 21 and April 21.) Respiratory problems and aches and pains would both have been more common if more winter months had been present in the sample. Conversely, gastrointestinal problems would have probably decreased in relative frequency had there been fewer summer man-months. Much of the large share of the All Other Problems category can be explained by the ninety-one injuries (55 percent of all injuries) treated by one VHW who worked in an area troubled by guerilla warfare.

Referring to table 3-3, it is encouraging to note that just over 75 percent of all the problems recorded by the VHW sample can be classified as prob-

Table 3-3
Patient Problems Recorded by VHWs

Problem	Definition	Number of Cases	Percentage of Cases	Seriousness[a]
1. Headache	Includes general body ache, muscular aches and pains, toothaches, earaches	246	9.8	NS
2. Eye problems	Except eye injuries	78	3.1	S
3. Pneumonia		20	0.8	S
4. Common cold	Includes "throat problems" that were probably sore throats	101	4.0	NS
5. Suspected tuberculosis	Includes cough (probably chronic) breathing problems, chest pain	34	1.4	S
6. Gastrointestinal problems	Includes abdominal pain, diarrhea, dysentery, vomiting, and worms	818	32.7	S
7. Weakness and anemia		344	13.8	S
8. Fever		309	12.4	S
9. Skin problems	Includes impetigo	42	1.7	S
10. Jaundice	"Yellow skin"	22	0.9	S
11. Injuries	Probably mostly lacerations and bullet wounds, many probably infected; excludes burns	164	6.6	S
12. Burns		22	0.9	S
13. Family planning		18	0.7	S
14. Injection		273	10.9	NS
15. Other problems	Deliveries (2), malnutrition (1), malaria (1), gonorrhea (1), broken bone (1), measles (1)	7	0.3	S
Total		2,498[b]	100.0	

[a] NS = problem probably not serious; S = problem potentially serious.
[b] VHWs had failed to record problems for 109 patients. Two problems were recorded for 108 patients. Three problems were recorded for 1 patient.

ably serious. They do appear to have been providing a valuable service to the rural population they served.

Table 3-5 presents the variety of services provided by VHWs with the relative frequencies of each in the period for which data are available. There appears to have been little demand for family-planning services from male VHWs, and in those services provided, an equal split occurs between oral contraceptives and condoms. Moreover, of all the treatments provided by VHWs, only penicillin might on rare occasions prove dangerous, but the

Table 3–4
Relative Frequency of Health Problems as Determined by a Rural Survey and From VHW Records
(percent)

Health Problem	Survey	VHW Records
1. Respiratory problems	18	7
2. Fevers	15	14
3. Gastrointestinal problems	26	37
4. Aches and pains	21	11
5. Eye problems	2	4
6. All other problems	18	27

Table 3–5
Relative Frequency of Treatments Provided by VHWs

			Patient Cost in Afghanis[a]	
Treatment	Number	Percentage	Adult	Child
Aspirin	583	21.5	4	3
Penicillin	137	5.1	22	13
Multivitamins	317	11.7	5	5
Oralyte	141	5.2	10	10
Iron	122	4.5	8	4
Piperazine	658	24.3	6	4
Tetracycline eye ointment	81	3.0	7	7
Sulfadimidine	89	3.3	6	
Oral contraceptives	9	0.3	2	
Condoms	9	0.3	2	
First aid	232	8.6	(5)	(5)
Nutrition education	1	0.0	0	
Referrals	48	1.8	0	0
Injection	280	10.3	(5)	(5)
Total	2,707	99.9		

[a]$1.00 equals approximately 40 Afghanis during the period in question.
Note: Costs given in parentheses are subject to the whim of individual VHWs; these were the charges recommended to the VHW.

amount of penicillin used by the VHWs in this sample does not appear excessive, just over 5 percent of the treatments provided. This limited experience appears to confirm the initial decision to provide VHWs with penicillin. The benefits almost certainly exceeded the risks involved.

Children's treatments were generally different only in the number of pills in the prescription, the exception being children's aspirin, which had nine 150-mg tablets per prescription compared with nine 500-mg tablets for adults. All VHWs were trained in how to provide medicines to very young children who might have trouble swallowing pills.

The information available is too limited to serve as a basis for evaluating the VHWs' skills in diagnosis, which are likely to be the major source of VHW error. Proper treatment for a given diagnosis, however, did not seem to be a problem. Frequent testing and informal discussions with the VHWs indicated that they learned and remembered the proper treatments for each medical problem.

In addition to the reasons for which curative services were sought and the treatments prescribed, the VHW's register book showed the date, the patient's name, his home village, and his age and sex. Data were collected from the register books of nine VHWs: two from Ghazni Province and seven from Paktia Province. Tables 3-6 and 3-7 examine the relationships between age, sex, and travel distance of 2,497 patients to these nine VHWs.

As can be seen from the right-hand columns in both tables, the majority or about 60 percent, of the VHW's patients had to walk less than 10 minutes to reach him. Seventy-eight percent came from within a 15-minute radius. The remaining 22 percent had to walk more than 15 minutes to reach the

Table 3-6
Distance Traveled by, and Sex of 2,497 VHW Patients

	Sex						
	Male		Female				
Distance (Minutes)[a]	Number	Percent[b]	Number	Percent[b]	No Information	Total	Percent[c]
0-5	494	70	216	30	10	720	40.7
6-10	236	67	118	33	0	354	20.0
11-15	213	70	93	30	0	306	17.3
16-30	151	75	51	25	1	203	11.5
31-60	43	63	25	37	0	68	3.8
> 60	90	76	28	24	0	118	6.7
No information	583	80	144	20	1	72.8	—
Total	1,810	73	675	27	12	2,497	100.0

[a] Minutes in walking time from patient's home village to VHW as estimated by VHW.
[b] Percentage figures exclude patients on whom no sex information was recorded.
[c] Percentage figures exclude patients on whom no distance information was recorded.

Table 3-7
Distance Traveled by, and Age Group of 2,497 VHW Patients

Distance (Minutes)[a]	AGE GROUP (years)								No Information	Total	Percent[c]
	0–4	Percent[b]	5–14	Percent[b]	15–44	Percent[b]	>44	Percent[b]			
0–5	108	15.2	167	23.5	331	46.6	104	14.6	10	720	40.7
6–10	43	12.1	67	18.9	198	55.9	46	13.0	0	354	20.0
11–15	33	10.8	56	18.3	179	58.5	38	12.4	0	306	17.3
16–30	37	18.2	42	20.7	90	44.3	34	16.7	0	203	11.5
31–60	11	16.2	23	33.8	27	39.7	7	10.3	0	68	3.8
> 60	19	16.1	19	16.1	72	61.0	8	6.8	0	118	6.7
No information	175	24.0	127	17.4	366	50.3	60	8.2	0	728	—
Total	426	17.1	501	20.1	1,263	50.8	297	11.9	10	2,497	100.0

[a] Minutes in walking time from patient's home village to VHW as estimated by VHW.
[b] Percent figures exclude patients on whom no age information was recorded.
[c] Percent figures exclude patients on whom no distance information was recorded.

VHW from their home village. Conversations with VHWs indicate that a significant fraction of these probably made the journey primarily for a non-medical reason.

The relatively limited geographic access to the VHW supports several of the program's design features. Since Afghanistan's population is quite widely scattered, the number of people served per VHW will be very limited. Large numbers of VHWs will be required to provide access to a majority of the rural population. Therefore, training should be minimized, focusing only on priority problems, in order to hold costs down. Similarly, VHWs should be part-time workers, since the number of people they serve is unlikely to support a full-time worker.

The bottom row of table 3–6 shows that nearly three-fourths of the VHWs' patients were males. This had been anticipated, and an initial attempt to recruit females for VHW training had eventually been dropped in favor of concentrating efforts on the specially designed *dai* training program, which included a large component of child care. In theory, once both VHWs and *dais* had been trained from the same geographic area, the *dais* could assist the VHW in the treatment of female patients.

There is no obvious association of the patient's sex with the distance traveled. One might guess that restricted female mobility in a traditional Muslim society would result in a larger percentage of female patients coming from shorter distances. This does not appear to have been the case.

The distribution of VHW patients by age shows that adults are overrepresented. While children aged 14 and under constitute about 50 percent of the total rural population, they received only 38.2 percent of the VHWs' services, as indicated by number of patient visits. The bias is probably greater than this comparison indicates. Because 50 percent of all deaths in Afghanistan occur in infants and children under 5, this segment of the population should account for a high percentage of VHW patient visits. However, this segment actually claims 17.1 percent, slightly less than its share of the total population, estimated to be about 18 percent. Had *dais* been trained from the same villages as VHWs, the proportion of child and infant patient visits might have increased through referrals from *dais* to VHWs.

Preventive Services: No hard data have been collected on the ability of Afghan VHWs to deliver preventive services. The evaluation survey of Jaghori Woleswali of Ghazni Province, scheduled for the summer of 1979, would have focused on this aspect of the VHW's work. However, the lack of any incentive system for VHWs to provide such services probably signals a major weakness in the VHW Program as implemented. There was first and foremost no financial support for the provision of preventive services. Villagers could not be expected to pay the costs because they did not perceive the need. For the government to have paid a salary to VHWs to do preventive work would have doomed the program to almost certain failure; the government's Basic Health Centers could not provide minimal preventive services to even the most limited catchment area despite relatively well-trained and salaried staff; the possibility of the government supporting and supervising preventive work by thousands of VHWs was beyond consideration.

Nevertheless, attempts were made to impress upon the VHW the importance of prevention. More than 50 percent of the training hours were devoted to preventive concepts and services. In particular, the VHWs were trained to discuss prevention with patients every time they appeared with a curative problem. There is no evidence that this service was not provided; the post-posttest scores cited earlier indicate that the VHWs had not forgotten what they had been taught.

It seems doubtful that the VHWs did much in the area of health education. In their first continuing-education program, the VHWs in Sarobi Woleswali designed a flipbook to be used in educating the villagers about the importance of clean drinking water. The printed flipbook was then distributed to the same VHWs at their second continuing-education course 6 months later. Political events at that time interfered with the course of the program, and no follow-up was made.

The management team tried, on a very small scale, to develop a village water-supply program to be associated with the VHW. In Sarobi Woleswali, Ministry sanitarians, who were paid incentive per diems by the management team, used UNICEF-provided materials and free labor donated by villagers (mobilized by the VHW) to construct piped gravity-flow drinking-water systems in two villages. Rough cost estimates indicated per capita costs competitive with more complex systems being implemented in market towns by the Ministry's Environmental Health Department.

Because of UNICEF opposition to the payment of incentive per diems, modified experiments were tried in Girishk Woleswali. Sanitarians made one trip to select sites for half a dozen wells; without the incentive, however, no follow-up visits were made, and a year later the wells had not been dug.

Acting independently, and on the basis of their training, the VHWs may have had some effect on village water supply. At least one VHW was observed to have improved the spring from which his family got its drinking water.

Primary Health-Care Development personnel observed that several VHWs constructed sanitary latrines after their training. These latrines were primarily for the use of the VHWs own household, and it is doubtful that they had any significant impact on the health of anyone else.

With the active cooperation of the vertically organized Expanded Immunization Program, the team assisted in an immunization experiment using VHWs. Largely owing to the efforts of an exceptionally motivated sanitarian at the Sarobi BHC, the experiment was quite successful. Sarobi VHWs received intensive training in the importance and practical techniques of immunization during a 3-day continuing-education session. The BHC was provided with an electric refrigerator, vaccines, and specially designed immunization cards with plastic envelopes to be kept by each child's parents. A register was maintained by the Village Health Worker. On a prearranged date, the BHC sanitarian brought vaccines (DPT, tetanus toxoid, measles, BCG, polio, and smallpox) to the village. The local VHW, working with members of the village health committee and other volunteers, would get the target population to a central location and would then help administer and record the vaccinations.

Both VHWs and villagers responded well. Rural people are generally favorably disposed to vaccinations because of the successful eradication of smallpox. During the following weeks, over a thousand vaccinations were administered. It was the first time that either measles or polio vaccine had been administered in a rural setting in Afghanistan. This has been possible, however, only because of the unusually motivated sanitarian in Sarobi. Without better-supported BHCs and additional incentives for workers, such an effort could not be expected to be sustained.

VHWs were trained in one other quasi-preventive activity: the detection of malnutrition among children using the nutrition arm band. There was no expectation that the VHW would systematically screen all children in his village, and except for multivitamins and iron tablets, he had to rely solely on health education as treatment. VHW effectiveness in nutrition was probably minimal, at least outside his own extended family.

In summary, then, very little information exists by which to evaluate the effectiveness of the VHW in the delivery of preventive services. Since the program design did not include specific incentives to encourage the delivery of these services, it may be presumed that the VHW had relatively little impact, except possibly in his own family.

VHW Patient Costs: Patient-visit costs are fairly easy to estimate from the information in table 3–5, which shows the treatments provided in 2,475 patient visits. The total cost of all drug prescriptions, assuming only adult prescriptions, would be 17,012 Afghanis, which, when reduced to account for child prescriptions, becomes 16,156 Afghanis. Assuming VHWs charged the recommended 5 Afghanis for injections and first-aid treatments, an additional patient cost of 2,560 Afghanis is incurred. The average patient-visit cost, then, works out to be 7.6 Afghanis, or approximately 19 cents.

For patients receiving drugs, the average cost was slightly higher: 8.4 Afghanis per patient visit, or about 21 cents. This compares favorably with the average cost of a visit to a pharmacy, as indicated by villagers in "A

Health Survey of Three Provinces of Afghanistan" (November 1977). There, the cost, including transportation, was 248 Afghanis, or approximately $6.20, nearly 30 times the cost of a VHW patient visit.

Three principal factors were responsible for the low cost of patient visits to VHWs. First, and probably most important, the VHW used generic drugs purchased via a revolving-fund mechanism through UNICEF at a small fraction of the cost of the brand-name drugs sold at pharmacies. Second, VHWs brought the drugs to the patients, minimizing patient travel costs. Third, the VHW's profit was only 2 Afghanis per prescription, accounting for only 26 percent of the cost to the patient; pharmacy markups are undoubtedly considerably greater. Fourth, the Ministry subsidized the cost of the logistics system by providing free transportation from Kabul to the BHC and by providing the salary of the storekeeper at the BHC.

Several other costs are not included in the preceding calculation. These are the program costs, that is, training costs, supervisory costs, start-up capital costs (cabinets, chairs, and other equipment all provided by UNICEF), and program-management costs. The magnitude of these costs is a little difficult to estimate, but preliminary calculations indicate that training and start-up costs amounted to about $400 per VHW. If this cost depreciated at 10 percent per year, and if one estimates the overhead costs (borne by the MOPH) at $60 per year per VHW, then the program costs amount to approximately $100 per year per VHW. Experience indicates that VHWs receive about 450 patient visits per year, yielding an average cost of 22 cents per patient visit, which is borne by the MOPH and foreign aid donors. The estimated total cost, then, is 19 cents (borne by the patient) plus 22 cents (borne by the government) to equal 41 cents per VHW patient visit.

Conclusion

The concept of Village Health Workers was new in Afghanistan when the program began and there were adjustments to be made on the part of Ministry officials, the management team, and villagers alike. Although the program was suspended by political turmoil before the anticipated levels of operation had been fully realized, certain observations can be made.

Prior to the VHW Program, the only regularly available providers of health care in Afghan villages were the indigenous practitioners. For certain ailments, most villagers clearly preferred "modern" medicine, which was available only at the nearest Basic Health Center or pharmacy, many located at prohibitive distances from their villages. From the villagers' point of view, there was a great need for a knowledgeable practitioner that lived right in their village and was available winter or summer, day or night.

The initial experience in training and supporting VHWs indicates that they can make an enormous psychological difference to remote village people. The VHW's certificate, framed neatly on the wall, reassures the villagers that the VHW training has meant something. The VHW's well-stocked drug cabinet within a 10-minute walk of most villagers means that when Mohammed Sadeq's son becomes suddenly sick and feverish at 3:00 A.M., there are effective "modern" remedies close at hand. The VHW's effect on village confidence and morale is positive, and it is perceived as a useful government contribution to the community.

Most villagers have minimal knowledge of, or appreciation for, preventive medicine and health education, but when they or their children are sick, they know what they want, and the VHW is a more than acceptable means of satisfying that want. The VHWs themselves responded enthusiastically to the new program as well. Many of them literally memorized their manuals during training, recognizing that this might be their only opportunity to become something more than an impoverished peasant. In the village, their new status gave them respect and prestige among their fellow villagers.

Unfortunately, the VHW Program was suspended prior to surviving long enough to test the notion of sustained village loyalty and support. Such loyalty toward government initiatives is not easily won in Afghanistan; there have been too many broken promises by well-dressed men from Kabul for the villager to be anything but skeptical. The bits of evidence that do exist point to increasing village support. It all takes time, a great deal of time. The government official has to visit the village many times, and he has to come through on his promises. The relationship between government and village is one of gradually developing reciprocal trust, and satisfactory progress in the VHW Program had led to Ministry and the team to be optimistic.

A significant exception followed from an effort to train a group of nomad health workers (NHWs) in March of 1978. The idea was discussed with nomads in Paktia Province; it was decided that they would be trained while they were grazing their flocks in Logar Province in the late spring. Despite the assurances of the Paktia nomad Khans, the NHW recruits did not meet in Logar at the agreed-on time. The fundamental problem was trust. Afghan nomads have kept their culture and way of life intact for centuries by avoiding all contact with government officials and government agencies. Despite the fact that a few progressive tribal Khans made a decision to participate in the program, and despite a profound felt need for NHWs (documented in a survey of Paktia nomads in February and March of 1978), the majority of nomads could not bring themselves to cooperate in a government-organized training program. The "April Revolution" of 1978 has since further reduced the level of trust in government of both nomads and villagers.

The current political situation in Afghanistan requires that judgment be suspended on the final result of the VHW Program effort. Since March of 1979, training, supervisory, and supply systems have all ceased. Nevertheless, surviving trained VHWs are continuing to perform the skills they have learned; the knowledge and skills passed to villagers cannot easily be taken from them.

C. The Development of the National *Dai* Training Program
John W. LeSar

Introduction

The National *Dai* Training Program has completed more than 2 years of activity since the first *dai* (traditional midwife) was trained in June of 1977. By June of 1979, over 540 *dais* were trained, and the program is expected to expand greatly if the political climate stabilizes. What is the history of the program? What has succeeded, what has failed, and why? What needs of the community has the program served to lead to widespread acceptance even in a turbulent period of Afghan politics? This section will try to answer these questions in order to illustrate how program planning, a newly designed curriculum, and rapid start-up have combined in the development of a nationally implemented program.

Demonstration of Need: Why a Dai Program?

The *dai* has been an important component of the indigenous health-care system in Afghanistan for centuries, attending deliveries and bringing health services and health education to women in the village setting. Because most Afghan women are confined to their homes or the homes of close relatives, the role of the *dai* in reaching them with health-related information is critically important and something that no man can do.

While the health-care system in Afghanistan is rapidly expanding, about 75 percent of births are still attended by the traditional village *dai* (15 percent by female family members and 10 percent by western-type practitioners). Since so much of Afghanistan's population is widely scattered in rural areas, health-care coverage of the population, although increasing, is not expected to be complete in the near future.

In 1977, there were 12.5 to 13 million rural people in Afghanistan, both settled villagers and nomads. At a growth rate of 2.5 percent per year, this segment of the population would be expected to reach 14.1 million to 14.7 million people within 5 years. While the MOPH hopes to have about 250

Basic Health Centers in operation by 1982, optimistically these will provide services to only about 2.5 million people (at a coverate rate of 10,000 people per BHC), leaving 11.6 million to 12.2 million rural people still without access to basic health services. Furthermore, although all BHCs are supposed to have female workers, only 29 percent do at the present time. Thus the gap in health services to rural women is even wider than that for the general population.

The *dai,* then, continues to be a critical resource in the village and offers promise as a significant contributor to a modern-day health system. The *dai* is a villager herself, whereas most better-trained health workers are more urban in background. Because the *dai* can relate to village women in their own cultural framework and through training can also relate to the health system, she can help the community accept new ideas and new medical treatments. Together, these traits make the *dai* a community health resource of considerable importance.

In the Ministry's decision to begin a *Dai* Training Program as a complementary alternative health-delivery strategy, a first step was to set goals and to calculate the need for trained *dais* in rural Afghanistan. To achieve coverage of 1,000 people per dai (50 to 60 pregnancies per year, about 200 children under age 5), about 11,000 *dais* would be needed. Alternatively, one *dai* for each village over 500 people suggested a need for 18,000 *dais.* Utilization of *dais* also was considered. At the present time, pregnant women usually prefer the *dai* to a female worker at the BHC, supporting wide utilization; on the other hand, if urban migration intensities, the utilization of *dais* might decrease. Thus it seemed safe to predict a need for at least 15,000 trained *dais.*

Program Development

Development of a Receptive Environment: The creation of a receptive environment within the Ministry of Public Health was crucial to the early development of the program and to its subsequent stabilization. Many factors helped create a low-risk situation for senior Ministry officials. The first was the demonstration of need. Other factors included the following: the *dais* were indigenous workers already functioning in the villages, and no existing health worker was directly threatened by the training of illiterate *dais* in rural areas; the international climate in health favored the development of primary health-care workers (village workers); there was no cost to the MOPH (USAID paid for the field test through its Basic Health Services contract); and the team assumed the role of risk takers in the initial testing of the program.

The role of outsiders as risk takers is often not well understood. Program failure can be blamed on the foreigners who misjudged the culture and its people. However, program success can be readily accepted by Ministry officials who not only allowed the program in the first place, but were smart enough to get international donors to pay for it. The team had consistent success in filling this role as part of a productive two-way relationship with the Ministry. Environmental preparation included

Achieving political legitimacy: Political legitimacy was achieved through the development of *dai* training as a research-and-development experiment closely associated with the management team. Once two small groups of *dais* had been trained and Ministry decision makers had observed the results, the government began to make public announcements about the program. Later, after the third class had finished training, donor interest and continued good results prompted the government to consider a national program, which was developed in the late fall of 1977. The Basic Health Services Department, the team, and United Nations Fund for Population Activities (UNFPA) became the main sponsors of the expanded National *Dai* Training Program of Afghanistan.

Gaining support of opinion leaders: The support of Ministry and donor decision makers was gained by their direct contact with the training program—usually at graduations when senior Ministry officials were speakers. In the rural areas, the *woleswal* (district governmental leader) encouraged village opinion leaders to support the program, who did so only moderately until the graduates returned home safely and villagers observed their new skills.

Obtaining trust and confidence: Trust and confidence were gained by producing quality graduates in the early programs, by the fact that the program leader was known to be an honest and responsible person, and by the team's credibility in the Ministry based on earlier performance. The team had extensive training experience with health workers; Afghans and donors felt secure that with continued team assistance, the quality of training and the management of the training function would improve, resulting in Ministry organizational competence over the project term. After the initial 6 months of the program, an Afghan advisor of known skills and management ability was hired, further building trust in the program and confidence in its success.

Securing initial funding: Funding for the experimental phase was by USAID through the management team contract. By the fifth month of the program, donor interest was high, and a cooperative and coordinated donor funding package was developed in the late fall of 1977.

This package allowed a rapid expansion of *dai* training at minimal expense to the government. Owing to continued low budget allocations for rural health services, this donor package was crucial to the development and sustenance of a receptive environment within the Ministry.

Donors were interested because the *Dai* Training Program was a village-centered approach to health development, a current major health policy thrust of WHO, UNICEF, and USAID. UNFPA also was broadening its mandate to include MCH services so the donor field staff had guidance that fit with the objectives of the *Dai* Program. The management team played an important role in developing the receptive environment that enabled the *Dai* Program to begin. The management team was able to coordinate the public information campaign and the project writing, which led to a program funded by three major donors: UNFPA, UNICEF, and USAID.

The first role of the team was in experimentation and as risk takers for the program during early field testing. The second role was the coordination of the public-information campaign. This was done mostly through planned visits to the field by various donor field and headquarters staff. *Dai* training was observed by UNICEF, UNFPA, and U.S. government personnel, including the American ambassador, all senior staff of USAID/Kabul, and two AID/Washington officials. By seeing the *dai* in action, these decision makers could see the potential of such a program in Afghanistan.

A third coordinating role was in program planning. Of the major donors, only USAID had a technical expert in public health on its staff. UNICEF and UNFPA program officers were generalists by background; technical program planning was therefore accomplished by the management team staff. Since Ministry personnel were not experienced in the type of program planning required by donors for submission to their headquarters, the team helped translate Ministry desires into donor-type programming as required.

A fourth coordinating role was the actual document writing. The team coordinated the document writing necessary for tripartite donor funding. This process was greatly facilitated by team personnel with project-writing experience in both UN and USAID formats. Document-writing skills are generally not found in Afghan health personnel, and it is unreasonable to expect that they should keep up with the jargon and convoluted formats that tend to emerge from bureaucracies.

Design of the Program: *Development of Organizational Objectives:* The *Dai* Training Program, at the start of the program in June of 1977, had the following objectives. *Dais* should:

Be recruited from rural villages and small towns and should be already recognized by their community;

Be trained to recognize normal cases from serious and nonserious cases;

Be trained to treat and give health education to normal and nonserious cases and to refer serious cases to the Basic Health Center or hospital;

Receive training in obstetrics, family planning, and child care for the under-five child as part of their basic course;

Receive remuneration for their services after training in the same ways as before their training;

Not require any special drugs or expendable supplies as a result of their training;

Receive continuing education at least yearly;

Be rigorously evaluated for skills development during their training and should be evaluated on these skills at each continuing-education session;

Have their performance observed in the village after training, and the opinions of the village women should be sought in evaluating *dai* performance;

Be encouraged to serve their people and their country.

By the time the effort had become expanded into a nationwide effort, more specific goals and objectives had been developed. The long-range goal was to reduce mortality, morbidity, pain, and suffering among village women and children and to give villagers choices about their family size by the training of village traditional midwives who would be part of an integrated maternal and child health-care system. Objectives for the first years of the program included:

Training not less than 3,500 *dais.*

Training the *dais* in the following skills:

Early detection of the high risk of pregnancy
Recognition of abnormal conditions of the postpartum period
High-quality treatment and health education of the normal pregnancy
Early detection of serious illness in the young child with prompt referral
Early detection of childhood malnutrition

Treatment of the child with nonserious illness
Health education for the child who is well or nonseriously ill
Family-planning education
Communication skills

Developing a program-management structure that can guarantee quality *dai* performance by a

High-quality basic training system
High-quality continuing-education system
Field-evaluation system

The objectives for the first year were to train not less than 450 *dais,* demonstrate high-quality training by good posttest scores, train and make operational five training teams, develop a training-team supervision program, develop field-evaluation procedures, and demonstrate continuing government and community acceptance of the program. The objectives, which were specific and easy to explain, guided the development of the support organization and facilitated evaluation by Ministry and donor decision makers.

Development of a Financial Plan: The financial plan for the first year, plus a tentative 5-year plan was developed by the team and the donor agencies. Detailed budgets were prepared for the costs of each training team and the costs of the program-management staff. Based on the first-year plan, a donor-government funding package was developed for $270,000.

An important facet of the team coordinating process was the development of "ownership" by each donor agency. The plan was developed in such a way that each donor funded specific parts, which allowed it to honestly claim the program to its headquarters. The resultant funding package for year one follows:

Percent Contribution by Donors
(Direct Program Costs)

UNFPA	55.7
UNICEF	25.7
USAID	13.3
GOA	5.4

In addition, USAID supported the program extensively through its ongoing contract. This included continued technical assistance, typing, financial coordination, bookkeeping, and loan of vehicles, drivers, and field supplies until UNICEF vehicles and supplies arrived. Thus, between June of 1977 (when the first *dais* were trained) and December of 1977, the international donor community was oriented, exposed to the objectives and methods of the program, assisted in project writing and development of a coordinated donor assistance plan, and had their plans accepted, in principle, by their headquarters. The result was a 5-year donor commitment to the National *Dai* Training Program.

Development of Internal Structure: The people working in the National *Dai* Training Program were organized as shown in figure 3–1. The program was one of four directorates of the Presidency of Basic Health Services, along with Basic Health Center Training and Supervision, Village Health Workers, and Administration.

In 1978, five coequal training teams, each headed by a nurse-midwife, were formed. Each nurse-midwife was assisted by two female health workers (high school graduates given special training by the *Dai* Training Program staff) and a trained *dai.* The *dai,* a graduate of the program, was given additional training in teaching methods, pregnancy, and child care and was an integral part of the training team.

The program-management section contained the director, a physician, a full-time UNFPA advisor, a team member's part-time assistance, two positions for physician-supervisors, two nurse-midwives for field evaluation, and one training-materials nurse. The physician-supervisor posts and only one of the nurse-evaluator positions were filled in the first year of the program, because start-up training activities occupied everyone's time. The technical aspects of training, evaluation design, and implementation are discussed in appendix E.

Program Evaluation

Factors in Leadership Acceptance: The effectiveness of the *dai* training organization was largely due to its leadership. Acceptance of this leadership rested both on personal attributes of the leaders and on organization of the leadership fucntions.

Personal Leadership Factors: It is important to understand how project leaders worked together to achieve program objectives. Early in the program, the President of Basic Health Services and the team provided the important political status that convinced the Minister to approve field testing. The training advisor provided the professional status early in the program, and personal commitment by program leaders has been strong and

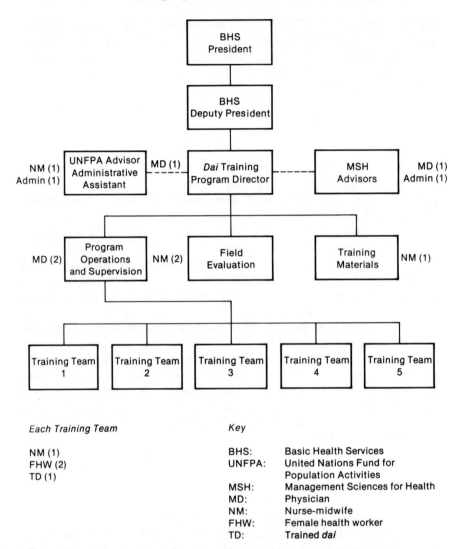

Figure 3-1. National Dai Training Program Organizational Chart

constant. This commitment has been vitally important in creating a close-knit organization and in maintaining momentum in an often turbulent environment.

Organizational Leadership Factors: The entire organization has grown significantly in terms of competence, so that the organization itself now has a leadership role in training methodology—not just in *dai* training, but in pedagogy, teacher training, and training evaluation. These skills are probably only matched by one other training organization within the Ministry. Leadership roles were distributed so that personal friction has been minimized. There are few competing roles; most are complementary and mutually supportive. This has been possible because of the personal attributes of the people selected by the director and the UNFPA advisor, plus good planning of the organizational structure.

Leadership Development: The team training advisor provided most of the early guidance for leadership development of *Dai* Program staff, with the Afghan UNFPA advisor assuming a key role in development of leadership within the *dai* organization after the first 6 months.

There has been an underlying personal-development philosophy that has guided the development of Afghan leaders in this program. This experiential-learning philosophy assumes that the best learning method is for people to experience, under supervision, the situations they will face in their jobs. A second premise is that until people experience the job situation, they are unable to make expert judgments about the correct ways to proceed in their jobs; theory is not enough. The application of this philosophy in the *Dai* Program is described in the following paragraphs.

At the beginning of the program, there was political pressure to start the program quickly. Owing to these circumstances, and the previously mentioned belief that the Afghans should experience one training methodology before making judgments about others, the team training advisor assumed an operational role in program management and also developed the curriculum. Short, nonformal training was provided for the director and two or three nurse-midwives in how to teach using the new curriculum. The first program trained about eleven *dais;* test scores and impressions of involved persons suggested that the program was an apparent success. The President of Basic Health Services and the team then developed the political support that allowed a second field test 2 months later. Operational control remained generally in the hands of the training advisor, but the director assumed responsibility for recruitment of *dais* and day-to-day supervision of the training. The Afghans and the team revised the curriculum. The training advisor remained present for almost all of the first two training classes, where he worked with the nurses on their teaching techniques and supervised the development of the practical aspects of the training. By the end of the second training program, the director and two or three nurse-midwives could do the training without supervision. The third *dai* training course was done without the training advisor's supervision.

After the third course, the UNFPA advisor was hired. By that time, the donor-assistance plan had been developed. At that time, approval of a plan using five training teams to train 450 *dais* in Afghan year 1357 (March 1978 to March 1979) seemed likely. The UNFPA advisor's initial tasks were to plan the next training program, supervise it, begin the recruitment of staff for the expanded program to begin 5 months later, and begin to coordinate donor-related activities. Beginning in December of 1977, the training advisor's time with the *Dai* Program decreased dramatically, and the director and UNFPA advisor began to assume program control.

At this point in time, the program was operated by Afghans. The team provided advice when asked and continued to contribute in technical areas where the staff still was uncertain (curriculum development, field evaluation, continuing education). However, the program decision makers were all Afghans.

Thus leadership development within the *Dai* Program of Afghanistan proceeded from initial control and guidance by the team, through supervised training and management control by Afghans, to complete decision-making control by Afghans. This step-by-step approach has developed Afghan capability in training and management through supervised experiential learning. Now the Afghan leaders are the experts. They can now experiment with other training and managment techniques and compare them with their past experiences. The program may change as these leaders become more sophisticated managers and trainers, but the changes will be based on experience and not theory.

In summary, the leadership of the National *Dai* Training Program has been strong and of critical importance in the development and stabilization of the program. The leaders themselves had inherent strengths that brought political status, professional status, technical competence, and commitment to the program. Organizational leadership within the MOPH was developed through planned sharing of responsibilities and continuity of leaders. A leadership-development program based on supervised experiential learning contributed to Afghan assumption of entire program leadership within the first 15 months of the program.

Securing and Training of Personnel: The *Dai* Program developed a teacher-training program that all teachers were required to attend before conducting their first training class. By the time the third *dai* training class ended in early January of 1978, the national expansion had been approved. Three months were set aside for development of the *dai* training-staff skills. In mid-January, *dai* staff and other ministry trainers underwent a 3-week course in critical training and management skills given by a team consultant. The course further developed skills in pedagogy and in fundamentals of learning. The staff also gained awareness of planning by objectives, which assisted them later in developing a 6-month work plan for the program.

After the critical training and management skills course, the Afghans themselves initiated further training of *dai* staff. By this time, the program had decided to use twelfth-grade graduate women and previously trained *dais* as *dai* trainers under the supervision of a nurse-midwife. They organized their own 8-week teacher training course with planning assistance from the team. By June of 1979, eight teams had been trained and become operational.

Development of a Fast Start-Up: The program benefited from a fast start-up phase, which allowed decision makers and donors to see the results of the training. Demonstration of the proficiency of the trained *dais* was essential for program acceptance. Proficiency was determined by test scores before and after the training program and, more important, by a series of field visits where senior health officials could directly question the *dais* and observe them interacting with pregnant women and small children. Seventy-four *dais* were graduated in the first 6 months of the program.

Village acceptance was demonstrated early. First of all, the *dais* greatly enjoyed the training, often their first schooling in any formal sense. Second, the *dai* graduation exercises attracted a great deal of interest from village leaders and rural political and governmental leaders. Third, the word of mouth information diffusion process was quite rapid considering the low population density and difficulties of travel. By the end of the second training program, political and health officials in various parts of the country had heard of the program. Within the medical community, many Basic Health Center doctors and provincial health officers became supporters of these attempts to upgrade a well-known village health provider. The village constituency was expressing itself through its officials; it became a status symbol in some areas if the village had a trained *dai*. Adjoining villages pressed their leaders for training of their *dais*.

Maintenance of Acceptable Performance: A fast start-up with good results is not enough to achieve stabilization of the program. Acceptable performance must be maintained not only in the first year, but for 2 to 3 years until a steady state is reached. Many factors are important in maintaining acceptable performance.

Consistency with Objectives: The original mandate was to provide the *dai* with the critical skills necessary to function effectively. The curriculum has had six revisions since the first training class, but the core skills remain the same—pregnancy care, postpartum care, family planning, and child care for the under-five child. In addition, the *dais* have been taught communication skills to improve their ability to gain information and to give information to their clients.

Stability of Outputs: The output of trained *dais* has been quite constant since the program's inception, even in the turbulent political environment of 1357 (1978). The outputs of the training program by quarter are shown in table 3-8. The program entered a higher production phase in 1357 because donor and MOPH funding became available. The objective for 1357 was 450 new graduates; 470 were trained.

Feasibility in Relation to Resources: It is important to mention that donor resources have paid over 95 percent of program costs thus far. The program seems successful, and donors seem willing to continue funding it. There is, in fact, interest in more rapid expansion. However, over the next 4 or 5 years, donors want to decrease their percentage contribution. At this point it is not clear whether the Ministry will raise the resources to continue the program at production levels necessary to provide almost all village women access to a trained *dai* if donors do decrease contributions.

Conformity with Expected Behavior: The leadership of the *Dai* Program has tried to keep the program in conformity with its stated mandate. The program management staff has kept decision makers informed about the program's progress through verbal and quarterly reports and has generally been meeting targets. Most important, the program has not tried to expand its mandate, which could create competition with other organizations.

The program leadership also has conformed socially by obeying local cultural norms. The rapid assumption of leadership by Afghans with much rural experience, particularly in operational areas, has kept the program aligned with rural social values. This has been especially important in protecting the privacy of women.

Consistency with the Goals and Targets of Society and Parent Organizations: Specific goals and objectives for care of women and children in rural areas were not clearly articulated at the time the program began; the *Dai* Program developed in parallel to an increasing awareness that the villagers themselves were a major resource and lacked education and awareness rather than intelligence. The villagers themselves already knew who was helpful and not helpful in the village and had found useful medical practitioners of various types within their own environments. Once the *Dai* Program had shown villagers that their values were respected, particularly concerning the seclusion of women, they readily consented to having the *dais* trained. The benefit was clear and in conformity with the goals of villagers themselves.

When the program began, the Ministry was undecided as to whether it was a good idea or not. Most of the staff had been trained in schools that were influenced by developed-country models with different problems. The

Table 3–8
Training-Program Outputs, by Quarter

Year	Quarter	Outputs
1,356	1	11
(March 21, 1977 to	2	24
March 20, 1978)	3	37
	4	0[a]
1,357	1	95
(March 21, 1978 to	2	116
March 20, 1979)	3	120
	4	139
		542

[a] Staff development training

doctors were very concerned about quality of care and, although they would not usually admit it, about competition and loss of prerogatives. However, international opinion favored trials of village workers, and the team was present to absorb the initial risk and provide the money, technical advice, and encouragement. Thus field trials were approved, and constituencies were developed.

Sensing Malfunctions and Taking Adaptive Actions: To maintain acceptable performance, the program had to sense and correct problems early. The *Dai* Program did this by responding to any complaints about a trained *dai,* investigating the complaint, and taking corrective action if necessary. In addition, the student-evaluation system of the *Dai* Program always had complete data on the skills of each graduate in a readily available form. If problems arose, the program managers could consult the personnel card and the *dai*'s test scores could be examined.

Finding an Organizational Niche: The *Dai* Program succeeded in developing the trust and confidence of decision makers, in dealing with competition, and in establishing good interorganizational relationships. While many factors played a role, it was not a random process, and several points may be noted.

Development of Organizational Relationships: In the development of the *Dai* Program, three main characteristics of the development of organizational relationships can be described: (1) vertical programming, (2) power strategy, and (3) low profile with other organizational units. Once the initial field tests were complete, there were various ways in which *dai* training on a national scale could have developed. One way was to maintain tight vertical management control over all training teams and not allow outside interference. Another way was to maintain loose management control and decentralize the training to other health units such as provincial hospitals and Basic Health Centers. A third way was to merge with other training units such as the Village Health Worker Program, Auxiliary Nurse-Midwife School, or the Public Health Institute. The program and advisory staff chose to maintain tight management control in the first 2 years of the program for three reasons: (1) to maintain the quality of the training process, (2) to maintain the momentum of the program, and (3) to enhance organizational development.

Extensive efforts were made to develop a quality training program, including a technically advanced curriculum and teaching process, careful supervision of the training itself, and a good teacher training program. In the first year of the program, other management methods could not ensure that quality could be maintained; the program staff felt that the early receptive environment of the *Dai* Program was based on easily discernible improved skills in these illiterate village women. For this reason, decentralization of the program as well as merger with the Village Health Worker Program were discouraged.

The *Dai* Program completed its initial field tests in June of 1977. By December of 1977, donor support for five training teams had been secured and the program was expanding rapidly. Program management and advisory staff felt that continued rapid expansion of quality training was important to stabilize the organization, and to solidify the concept of *dai* training before competition became intense. Tight management control was seen as the appropriate expansion strategy.

A third reason for the tight vertical management-control strategy with training teams based in Kabul was to continue to develop organizational structure of the National *Dai* Training Program. In the first year, the organizational structure was weak, and long-term viability was not ensured. By continuing to develop the staff, organizational competence increased. This became evident to decision makers within the MOPH and increased the chances for the program to achieve its training objectives and to guarantee itself a leading role in future years when another management strategy might be appropriate.

Power Strategy: Strategies for social change can be divided into three types: power strategies, persuasive strategies, and educative strategies. Early development of the National *Dai* Training Program used a simple power strategy through control of resources to survive and grow. In this sense, it was a typical experimental program working in a controlled environment.

Once the initial field testing was completed, the early successes of the program brought vested interests to life, with subtle but real power battles occurring during the first 12 months of the project. During the first 6 months, these battles were mostly over program control, as people closely affected by the project sought to turn the successes their way. Although the program tried to find a wide base of support within the Ministry, this was difficult in the Afghan context. The program was sought by the Presidency of Nursing, the General President of Health Affairs (number three ranking member in the Ministry), and the director of the other major village program within the MOPH. The President of Basic Health Services and his supporters played a critical role in program stabilization. Using a power strategy based on successful development, control of funding of key parts of the program, and access to and influence with international donors, the President of Basic Health Services kept the program in its original position within the Ministry and kept it independent so that it could grow, stabilize itself, and develop its own constituency through steady, high-quality performance.

After the first 6 months, the program was fairly stabilized in its leadership. The next problems arose with outside vested interests who tried to alter program objectives and create rival training organizations. Through careful public relations, the Minister prevented such vested interests as practicing obstetricians and nurse-midwives from feeling very threatened by the program.

With this is mind, the President of Basic Health Services and his advisors played crucial roles in guiding the program through its initial years. Through leverage and prestige, the existing training organization has been protected. After 1 or 2 more years—when the infant program has grown up—widespread development of *dai* training organizations should be in the country's interest. At that time, the parent organization will then be able to play the coordinating and quality-control role necessary for other groups to do the training successfully.

Low Profile with Other Organizational Units: In the first 2 years of the *Dai* Program, steady organizational development has occurred and a receptive environment still exists. Using a vertical programming approach with tight management control and a power strategy when necessary, program personnel have protected the organization.

The third means of continuing this momentum was by maintaining a low profile compared with other organization units. This has been accomplished in the following ways. The rural areas where *dais* were trained had few organizational units of any kind, hence few competitors. Key decision makers in the MOPH were identified, and decisions were made only through them. Information given out about the *Dai* Program was carefully planned so that sufficient, yet not excessive, amounts of information were available. Other organizational units were given information and help when they requested it, but they were not flooded with unsolicited material.

One of the most precarious aspects of new program development and stabilization is potential encroachment on the role of existing workers. New programs are very fragile; vested interest groups can quickly bring great pressure to bear, and this usually affects the receptive environment and, subsequently, the enabling relationships necessary for program stabilization. The *Dai* Program did not affect the jobs or status of any government worker in rural areas. Hence competition with existing workers was avoided.

Some Lessons from the Dai Program

Although the Afghan *Dai* Program has been relatively successful, it may be instructive to review aspects of the program that were less successful in order to see if any useful lessons can be drawn.

The Difficulty of Maintaining Practical, "Hands-On" Training: The *dai* curriculum is based on the concept that learning is most effective and lasting when the student actually experiences during training that which he or she will be doing later. In the case of prenatal care, young-child care, and health education, it is essential that the *dai* learn by examining, treating, and educating women and children (under supervision). The *dai* training teams were themselves trained in these teaching methods.

Despite every effort by the central organization to keep the training practical, several training teams began doing less and less "hands-on" teaching and instead did more didactic teaching. Afghans have traditionally learned by memorization; the new teaching techniques were unfamiliar, and when out in the field and away from supervisors, the *dai* trainers were tempted to teach according to more familiar ways. Another reason for the shift in teaching methods had to do with traditional Afghan sex-role behavior. Nurse-midwives who headed training teams were often reluctant to take an active role vis-à-vis the health-center doctor in setting up clinical teaching arrangements so that the *dais* could learn from patients rather than on models or through role playing. As a result, more recent *dai* training courses have not provided very much patient contact for the *dais*.

The obvious lesson to be drawn from this experience is that frequent supervision of the *dai* trainers is necesssary, as well as regular continuing education. A curriculum, no matter how well designed, does not teach itself; cultural values and practices will affect teaching and training, so old habits die hard.

The *Dais*, No Matter How Well Trained, Are Part of a Larger Health System; Their Overall Effectiveness Depends on the Level of Functioning of that System: One important job of the trained *dai* is to refer problem cases and high-rise pregnant women to a doctor (in the BHC or hospital). The *dai* also refers seriously ill children to the health center. Unfortunately, the BHC doctors in Afghanistan are often ill-prepared to take care of high-risk pregnant women; in fact, most BHC doctors are less experienced and knowledgeable about delivering babies than the average *dai*. When a *dai* refers a pregnant woman to the BHC and she is not treated properly, the value of the *dai*'s screening and surveillance function is greatly reduced.

The lesson here is very simple. Any village-based program that depends on referral to higher levels of care must be sure that those higher levels can actually do the job. If not, the villager worker is rendered much less effective.

The Difficulty Involved in Trying to Change the Way *Dais* Practice Midwifery in the Village: Most of the Afghan *dais* who have been trained have been practicing midwives for 10 to 30 years. A 5-week course, no matter how well planned and organized, cannot easily change basic habits in such areas as hygiene, delivery techniques, or infant feeding practices. The *dais* can learn all that their trainers want them to learn; but when back in their village, how much have they really changed in practice?

This vital question, however, is extraordinarily difficult to answer under present circumstances in Afghanistan. With unrest in rural areas, evaluation teams have not been able to directly observe *dais* in the field. There is little doubt that a 5-week intensive course has some effect; what cannot be answered is how great this effect is.

The lesson here can perhaps be expressed best in terms of a dilemma. If village-level health workers are recruited among existing practitioners such as *dais,* barbers, or herbalists, certain well-established habits will be difficult to change. However, if people who are not indigenous practitioners are recruited, they are likely to receive less respect from fellow villagers and, at the same time, are at risk of threatening established health practitioners such as doctors. The health-center physician is probably less threatened by an established practitioner whose skills have been upgraded than he is by a totally new individual whose role and status in the village are much less clearly defined.

There is no best general solution to this problem. Each country that embarks on the road to improved village health must make its own choices and set its own priorities. The only universal generalization is that the more the villagers take part in the decisions, the more likely the program is to be accepted and the better off everyone is.

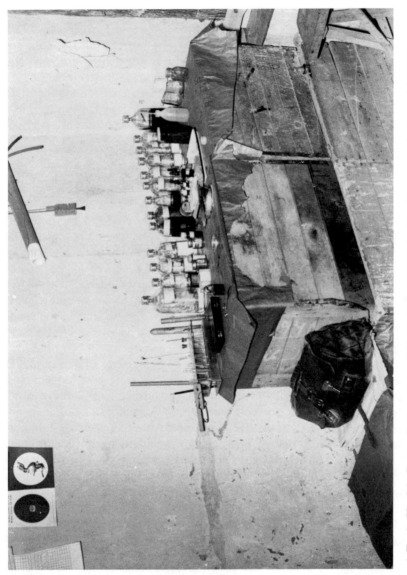

A Basic Health Center Laboratory. This is the only lab facility for a population of 50,000 people. Because of shortages of trained personnel, many such labs are not functioning.

Making Plans Happen: Central-Management Support Systems

Jerry M. Russell

A. Support Needs of the Field Program and Constraints in Meeting Those Needs

Field programs that provide direct services to the public on a national basis can be implemented and operated only to the extent that necessary support services—the routine management activities that ensure that the field programs have the personnel, materials, and finances required to function properly—are provided. In most cases, this is a central-government responsibility.

If the Afghan experience is any guide, the management of support services is the most difficult area of field program implementation in developing countries. No matter how admirable the objectives, how idealistic the planners, and how superior the preparation of the health workers, without support services the workers cannot be expected to make the programs succeed.

Many constraints contributed to the difficulties experienced in providing support services for rural programs in the Basic Health Centers, for the village health workers, and for the *Dai* Training Program. The constraints were not always the same in each of these field programs, reflecting differences in program complexity. For example, the program requiring the fewest support services, the *Dai* Training Program, experienced the fewest difficulties with support-service management. The following subsections examine three categories of constraints—personnel, organizational, and environmental—that the team encountered in assisting the Ministry in the development of management-support systems. Perhaps these constraints are not universal, but it is likely that they exist to varying degrees in all national programs in developing countries.

Personnel Constraints

Lack of Basic Preemployment or Preservice Management-Education and Training: Afghanistan has very limited management-education opportunities, and the few college graduates with this training go into either the private sector or the more prestigious Ministries, such as Finance,

Commerce, Planning, Mines and Industries, Foreign Affairs, or Interior. The high schools do not offer courses in this area, and even secretarial training is available to only a few students. Consequently, the Ministry was unable to recruit personnel who already had basic management and administrative skills. The Department of Administration, in fact, had only two college graduates among its own personnel. Most senior personnel in the Ministry were physicians, and most administrative staff were high school graduates with additional training. In order to recruit personnel with pre-existing skills, the Ministry had to tap experienced staff from other Ministries. New personnel seldom know how to do more than their supervisors were able to tell them, and the supervisors know only traditional procedures acquired by experience. Virtually no one had the broad management perspective required to plan, organize, direct, coordinate, and evaluate routine support systems, and few appreciated their importance.

Absence of Coordinated In-Service Training: There was no unit responsible for planning and implementing in-service training for either new or old employees of the Ministry. In-service training occurred on an ad hoc basis and largely ignored management training. New physicians assigned to Basic Health Centers might receive a brief preservice orientation that provided some information on the organization and regulations of the MOPH, their supporting responsibilities, and the benefits/requirements of civil service employment. There was no training in administrative skills or management concepts. The director of the Planning Department statistics section ran a basic mathematics course for his own staff; there were required but poorly attended Pashtu language classes for all government personnel; and some of the MOPH technical training schools, such as the Laboratory Technician School and the Auxiliary Nurse-Midwife School, held an occasional refresher course for their graduates. For clerical and other non-health-profession support staff, there was no training at all.

Inadequate Supervision: Supervision throughout the MOPH was an ill-defined concept and an even less-developed skill. Work-attendance records were checked, and personnel were reprimanded for poor attendance. Reprimands for poor work were known to occur, although there were no formal standards for judging work performance. Except in the vertical programs, such as the malaria program, supervision was never incorporated into routine visits with specific content. Seldom did the supervisors understand or pay attention to the administrative or organizational skills of those being supervised. Attention was much more likely to focus on attendance, the list of property signed out, or the general cleanliness of the room or building. Employees were occasionally punished if fault was found, but they were seldom recognized for doing a good job. Promotion was based on seniority, not performance.

Organizational and Structural Constraints

Structural Patterns Are National: The Ministry was virtually precluded from altering inefficient structures, and this reflected general government organization. For example, the Ministry Planning Department was responsible for construction and the capital-development budget activities. The budget section, responsible for annual or operational budgeting, was located within the Administration Department, and no one was responsible for seeing that the annual operating budget and development plans were compatible and mutually feasible. Plans for hospital construction, for example, occurred independently of any projections of future operational-budget requirements or availability.

Regulations and Procedures Are National: The Ministry was also subject to the same regulations and procedures as other agencies of the government. For example, the Ministry of Finance had budget, accounting, and warehousing manuals that all Ministries were expected to use. When these were found to be inappropriate, supplementary MOPH regulations would survive only as long as the person who introduced them was in a position of authority to enforce them.

Lack of Formal Job Descriptions and Operational Manuals: The first units within the MOPH to have detailed job descriptions were those assisted by the team, that is, Basic Health Center personnel, warehouse personnel, *dai* trainers, and village health workers. Other MOPH personnel did not have job descriptions by which they could be trained, by which their work could be judged, and by which they could be supervised. In addition, the various departments and offices had neither procedural manuals nor clearly defined objectives. Although some senior officials wanted such regulations to be developed, those at lower levels often appeared to resist, believing perhaps correctly that they could not be held accountable for that which has not been specified as their responsibility.

Environmental Constraints

Personal Economics: Although the Ministry received only a small portion of the government's budget, the lack of funds was not the major economic constraint to development of adequate support systems. In a country where the per capita annual gross national product is less than $200, where there is no social security other than the family, and where there are few jobs that provide the fringe benefits of government employment, civil servants are realistically reluctant to risk personal liability by making quick or generous decisions with valuable resources. An incorrect decision may result in loss of employment, personal liability for repayment, or even imprisonment. It is commonplace to encounter former civil servants, several years out of government service, still answering inquiries regarding money or property for which they were once responsible. As another example, the transfer of equipment or drugs from the Ministry's central warehouse to a Basic Health Center required a minimum of eleven signatures laboriously obtained. The bureaucracy provided security and release from personal liability at the price of inadequate field program support.

Tradition: Closely linked to the personal economic constraints are traditional practices that interfere with deployment of support services, protecting resources rather than dispersing them. All property, for example, is assigned to a trustee who has personal liability for it until it is formally transferred to another person. Every storeroom has a storekeeper, or *tawildar,* who has the only key to the padlock on the door. If he is absent, the storeroom can only be opened by a committee of three who must each sign a record showing exactly what was removed from the storeroom. On personnel matters, the traditional practice is to have a committee meet periodically to recommend decisions to the Minister. This practice is designed to limit favoritism or bribery, although, in practice, both could occur frequently. Elaborate procedures have evolved to ensure against the misuse of funds, procedures involving committees, numerous signatures, and several departments. The purchase of a tin of kerosene routinely takes three people half a day to accomplish. In all matters, but particularly those regarding physical or monetary resources, individuals refuse to take responsibility without the signature of their superior. With only senior personnel making decisions, relatively few decisions are made and relatively few resources are transferred or released.

External Constraints: In addition to constraints within the MOPH, external services and resources reflect the constraints of the Afghan environment. Mail from remote provinces frequently takes a month or longer to reach Kabul. None of the Basic Health Centers have telephones; they had to be contacted through provincial or district-level government offices. Ministry transport capacity is limited, and commercial carriers prefer to remain on the main roads where there is less damage to vehicles and some hope of return freight loads. They do not compete vigorously to take shipments to remote health centers. Roads into many mountainous regions are poor at best and are closed completely during winter snows and spring floods, which sometimes last 3 to 5 months. Bus service reaches most areas of the country, but road and weather conditions often make a trip to Kabul a 5-day journey. Basic Health Centers usually have a vehicle assigned to them, but since repair services and parts can only be obtained in the larger provincial cities, if at all, vehicles often sit unused for much of the year.

Conclusion

Combinations of constraints could easily be used to rationalize lack of effort to improve the central support systems discussed in this chapter. The professionally tempting approach of developing completely new support systems that might not be compatible with the overall structures of the government, that did not deal with the constraining realities of the country, or that could not be continued without foreign advisory assistance had to be avoided. The job was not one of designing new vehicles, but of making existing ones run a bit better.

B. Manpower Development: Formal and On-the-Job Training

Perhaps the most critical central-management support system deals with the development of human resources. Programs cannot exist without personnel, and personnel must be educated, recruited, oriented, and assigned to jobs. Ideally, a manpower-development system requires (1) job analysis and projections of manpower needs, (2) planning for the training and acquisition of personnel with the required knowledge and skills, (3) preemployment general and technical education, and (4) in-service training (continuing education).

Manpower development through the nearly 6 years of team work continued to be uncoordinated and largely unplanned, and it received many words, but low priority, on Ministry agendas. There was no focus of need analysis or planning and implementation of manpower-development programs. Need analysis was conducted by the program managers on an annual basis as part of budget preparation, an unsystematic process of accretion. There was no functional analysis of their programs, no job analysis of existing or planned positions, and no justification of positions approved in previous budgets.

A great handicap was the lack of control over, or significant input to, the major manpower training programs: medical schools and nursing schools. Both the medical schools and most of the nursing schools were under the Ministry of Higher Education, used traditional hospital-oriented curricula with virtually no public-health orientation and no health-management courses, and included little experience that would prepare students for the jobs they would have in Basic Health Services. The Ministry of Health did control the schools for sanitarians, laboratory technicians, and auxiliary nurse-midwives (ANM). Only the ANM school, with assistance from USAID, designed its curriculum to prepare students for work in the Basic Health Centers.

Although thwarted by the April 1978 revolution, donors, the Ministry, and the team had agreed on a phased manpower-development strategy that was incorporated in the 7-year health plan adopted the previous year. An analysis phase defining needs and resources requirements would precede establishment of a health-manpower institute. The Ministry conceived this to be a separate entity to circumvent the inertia and dead weight of the existing Public Health Institute, which on paper would appear to be the appropriate focus for such work.

Although a coherent manpower-development plan has never been implemented in the Ministry, Basic Health Services did make some progress in the form of analysis, planning, and training activities. Based on the Parwan-Kapisa Pilot Project, the team and the Ministry analyzed the functions of the Basic Health Centers, performed a job analysis of the BHC personnel, developed job descriptions, helped prepare operational manuals for the BHC staff, and assisted in the development and implementation of a mobile-team training program. Training activities included teaching trainers courses, preservice orientation for new doctors, continuing-education courses in technical areas, and administration of a foreign-training fellowship program that included both nondegree and degree programs in the United States and other countries. At the time of the April 1978 revolution, the first of four regional training centers was being opened, as noted in chapter 2.

The first manpower analysis in 1977 indicated that the Ministry had over 4,000 health service personnel. Many of these, particularly the physicians, were spending much of their time in management tasks. In addition, there were approximately 3,000 additional employees, including senior and mid-level managers, clerks, drivers, storekeepers, warehousemen, accountants, and support-service staff. For this latter group, there was virtually no other training available, either during employment or before. The Ministry had to rely almost completely on high school graduates who learned their jobs as they went along. Previous attempts to establish administrative training programs for civil servants had reached few people beyond the Ministries in which the programs were located, that is, Finance and Mines and Industries. With help from the team, the Ministry of Health developed a plan for an administrative training program to be implemented during the 7-year plan adopted in 1977. It was abolished by the new government in 1978.

C. Logistics System

Among management-support systems, logistics systems are of special interest because of the immediate disabling impact of inadequate supplies. This is manifested by (1) underutilization of facilities when medications are unavailable, (2) poor morale of personnel obliged to go through the motions without sufficient supplies, and (3) the premature termination of new programs before adequate testing or stabilization.

Although the team worked for 6 years in the area of logistics, it was not until the fourth year (1977) that the Ministry began to take concrete steps toward establishing a coordinated logistical system. The history of this slow, but persistent progress illustrates both the difficulties and possibilities in this critical area of health-organization development.

Central Warehouse

The original team contract provided for technical assistance in warehouse operations. When the team arrived in late 1973, the Ministry was in the process of constructing, with USAID support, a new central warehouse. Prior to that time, there were a number of smaller stores for drugs, supplies, and equipment scattered around Kabul.

The team analyzed the government's general warehouse regulations, the specific requirements of the Ministry, and then helped to develop a warehouse operations manual compatible with government regulations. The team assisted the Ministry in printing the necessary warehouse forms and file cards, obtaining adequate filing cabinets and training warehouse staff in the new warehouse procedures and record system. The team provided advisory assistance that gradually tapered off over the first 5 years of the project. In sum, it can be said that the warehouse-development assistance was successful. The new system continues in use. Drugs, supplies, and equipment were received, recorded, safely stored, and dispatched in an orderly manner. However, there were many problems and lessons to be learned.

A continuing problem was the frequent turnover of key warehouse personnel. During 1977 alone, there were four changes in the position of warehouse director. The team had provided warehouse training for the first director in the United States. He was then hired from the Ministry by UNICEF to handle their commodity imports because he was the only trained warehouseman in Afghanistan who knew something about health. Fortunately, there was less turnover among the lower-level warehouse staff. Although there was no continuity in direction, the overall warehouse procedures continued to operate reasonably well, which underscores the importance of instituting *systems,* not simply training individuals.

Another problem that hampered effective warehouse operations was the traditional Afghan storekeeper, the *tawildar*, who was assigned all property as a financially bonded storekeeper. If anything became lost, he was financially responsible. This led to the practice of padlocking all storerooms and not allowing anyone but the storekeeper to open them. If the storekeeper was absent, nothing could leave the storeroom, a practice that is not likely to change until the per capita income rises considerably and commodities are relatively less valuable.

A third major problem was the difficulty of maintaining adequate supervision. The training program and warehouse manual specify the need for goal-oriented supervision and assigned it to specific staff members. However, in practice, tradition often prevailed and supervisory practice reverted to checking for the presence of all assigned property, ad hoc assignments of the nearest person to the problem of the moment, and admonishments to subordinates when senior officials came to visit.

Thus, although supplies were received, stored, and dispatched, there was still much to do to improve warehouse operations. Perhaps the most important area needing improvement was the overall logistics system, of which the warehouse was but one important subsystem.

Logistics Management

From the beginning of its work in the Ministry, the team was involved in logistics management apart from the warehouse. Basic Health Services was actively standardizing the drug and equipment lists for rural health centers based initially on drug-use data and disease patterns in the Parwan-Kapita Pilot Project. The lists were then modified as more experience was gained in other regions of Afghanistan. In the Village Health Worker program, the team helped establish a functioning drug procurement, storage, repackaging, transport, and payment scheme.

However, it was not until the head of the Administration Department returned from 9 months of study in the United States that a full-time team member was acceptable and available to work as his counterpart. This is important, for most of the core offices in the logistics system were in the Administration Department: budgeting, purchasing, warehouse, and transport in particular. Much of the team advisor's work in the first year in the Administration Department was in helping the director develop a 5-year development plan.

In this process, considerable effort was spent in helping the director and other key Ministry officials approach management problems in a systematic way. The importance of this process cannot be overstated, for the traditional approach to management was crisis intervention with ad hoc solutions. The solutions usually consisted of placing blame on individuals and either reprimanding them or replacing them. The team cannot claim to have abolished this approach, but a few senior Ministry officials were beginning to see how they could use system analysis and planning tools to produce more lasting solutions.

The area of logistics is a good example. By the fall of 1977, the team was asked to provide a full-time logistics consultant. His first task was to map the existing logistics system. From this process, problem areas were identified and solutions were proposed. The major problem areas identified were poor communication links between components of the logistics system, and inadequate record and information system, piecemeal needs analysis and planning, and a lack of coordination. There were no overall guidelines for the logistics system, and only basic regulations existed for each of the offices involved. The linkages between the central logistics system and the technical health services departments were particularly poorly developed.

In late 1977, a new medical-supplies office was established to provide central coordination and action on logistics. By the fall of 1978, a comprehensive logistics operational manual was prepared, using the existing system to the maximum and adding only the important missing elements required to facilitate coordination. Unfortunately, the government changed at this time, the head of administration was replaced, and the logistics consultant's visa was not renewed. Had the logistics development program not been precipitously terminated, the process of training and the stabilization of the program would have been completed in an additional 2 years.

In conclusion, the Parwan-Kapisa Pilot Project showed the Ministry that clinic utilization tripled when an adequate supply of drugs was made available. Only a well-planned and coordinated logistics system can accomplish this on a regular basis. Beginning with a focus on the specific problems recognized initially by the Ministry, the team, the ministry, and the donors worked through a process of increasing awareness of broader logistics-management issues. In Afghanistan, this technical-assistance process in logistics took 6 years and was likely to have taken another 2 to 4 years before the system reached a stage of steady-state operations.

D. Management Information Systems

The Team and the Ministry worked on a wide variety of information systems over the 6-year period, from the extremely simple home-visit reporting system for use by illiterate trained *dais* to comprehensive information systems designed as the core of logistics management. These included information systems for the warehouse, mobile training teams, Basic Health

Centers, personnel management, financial management, village health workers, *Dai* Training Program, drug procurement, and others. Summary descriptions of some of these are included in this book, while more detailed presentations are contained in other MSH publications. Therefore, rather than reiterating what has already been presented, this section will describe some of the general problems and pitfalls experienced in planning and implementing information systems in Afghanistan.

The common problems encountered in information systems are the information does not come, that it is late, that it is incomplete, that it is inaccurate, that it is not analyzed, that it is not disseminated, that it is inappropriate, or that it is not used. There are several related reasons for this situation. Information-systems designers often design *data-production* systems rather than *management information* systems. The former produce data, perhaps of high quality, without regard to their relevance to the information needs of the organization's managers or their ability to use them. The latter approach attempts to provide the information managers require to make the best possible decisions in the time available. If design does not begin by asking what decisions the managers make and what information those decisions require, decision-oriented information systems are seldom produced.

Lest information-system specialists be given all the blame, it must be pointed out that they can carry out only the task given to them. Donor agencies frequently recommend or even require that the recipient organization develop something called a "health-information system," which usually refers to a system for collecting and analyzing data relating to indexes of the health status of a population and of the health services provided to that population. It seldom includes the routine organizational, financial, and personnel-performance data important for supervision, budgeting, training, and management support.

Another major problem with the use of information systems is *inadequate training*. Many people involved in technical assistance assume that decision makers will take appropriate action if they have accurate information. The fact is that the recipients of the analyzed data may know neither *how* to interpret them, nor *what* management decisions they should make from them. Everyone involved in the information system must be trained, including those who generate the data; those who collect, tabulate, and analyze them, and those who ultimately receive them. Stress is often placed on training the operators of the information system rather than the users of the information.

The opportunity to design and implement a completely new program (and the information system to support it) that does not involve preexisting personnel, regulations, and organizational traditions is rare. More commonly, the task is to make an existing program or organization function better. A revised information system is something that must be integrated into an existing structure. This means that the tasks, attitudes, and behavior patterns of staff must be altered, and training or retraining becomes the key to making the new information system work.

It is important to recognize that information systems already exist in every operational program. It may not be obvious to the outside observer, but the decision makers are already receiving and using information. The old system may not involve typed reports and quantifiable data, but the systems are there. The data include information about what one's superiors want, what is politically acceptable, the families of one's colleagues, what has been tried before, the attitudes and behavior of particular population groups, and the skills and attitudes of staff.

The lesson here, of course, is *not to assume* that organizational decisions are made solely, or even primarily, on the basis of information related to achievement of publicly stated objectives. Every organization devotes a significant proportion of its resources and time to that most basic of all objectives: survival. Every individual and department within the organization is concerned with his or its own survival. The more limited the resources and the more unstable the environment, the more prominent issues of survival in an organization will become.

Designers of information systems should consider how to analyze and present the information in such a way as to be useful to the organization's managers as they compete for an appropriate share of the organizations's and the country's resources. For example, data concerning population coverage of a program may be more *politically* important than data concerning the impact of the program on reduced morbidity or mortality. Data concerning comparative program costs and changes in costs are particularly useful. Managers want data that help their programs and organizations get an equitable share of resources.

E. Financial System

Four basic functions of financial systems are revenue generation, management of cash flow, budgetary control, and the production of data required for planning. The financial system used by the Ministry concentrated primarily on cash flow and budgetary control, with some attention to revenue generation and virtually no attention to planning. As with administrative systems, the financial system was the standard prescribed for all ministries and was not amenable to alteration by any single Ministry. Therefore, the team was restricted to two complementary approaches: helping to make the existing system operate better and helping to instiute modifications that would help the Ministry without conflicting with the standard government requirements.

Revenue Generation

All money used by the Ministry came to it from or through the Ministry of Finance, which obtains funds from taxes and donor-agency contributions. The Health Ministry could influence the amount it received through negotiations with donor agencies (USAID, WHO, UNICEF, and FAO) and through annual budget submissions to the Cabinet. Fees collected from patients for such items as x-rays, private rooms, and laboratory services went to the Ministry of Finance and did not increase the health budget. Money received from the sale of drugs through government pharmacies and to private pharmacies went back to the government's semiautonomous Avicenna Pharmaceutical Institute, beyond the Ministry's direct control.

Neither the budget section in the Department of Administration nor the planning section in the Department of Planning was able to examine potential benefits or project long-range cost implications of specific plans. As an interim measure, the team worked with the Ministry in preparing both annual budget submissions and budgets for multiyear development plans. In 1977, two publications were prepared for, and used by, the Ministry in preparing its budget. The *Financial Analysis of Health Programs* was essentially a cost-benefit study of existing and planned health programs (see appendix C). It was used by the Ministry in the development of its 7-year plan, by focusing attention on the potential productivity of alternative investments of the limited resources available. A second publication, *Financial Projections for the Ministry of Public Health,* analyzed the discrepancies between the development plans, which were primarily construction efforts, and the money potentially available to operate these facilities. The Ministry used these projections to revise its plans and to negotiate with the Planning and Finance Ministries for more realistic operational budgets. For the 1978 budget, for example, the Ministry of Finance set a ceiling of 7 percent increase over the 1977 levels for the entire government, but based on the case made by the Ministry, health was given a 12.38 percent increase.

Based on this positive experience with financial analysis, the Ministry established a financial-analysis office in the Department of Administration, which in turn established provincial financial-data units beginning in 1978. Although the "April Revolution" precluded this plan from progressing, the experience illustrates one way by which consultant assistance can lead to the institutionalization of new systems or subsystems.

The Ministry and the team, with USAID encouragement, also worked closely on another major area of revenue generation: obtaining donor assistance. The team was frequently able to help bring the Ministry needs to the attention of donor agencies in a form that could be acted upon, as discussed in chapter 5.

One area of revenue generation in which concrete assistance was provided related to pharmaceuticals. The rural surveys indicated that in 1976, Afghans spent approximately 6.9 billion Afghanis privately for drugs and health care, more than 10 times the government's expenditure. In the *Financial Projections,* the team called attention to this potential source of revenue and recommended that the Ministry should tap it through drug sales and other fees. The Village Health Worker Program became the first to develop and implement a system for prepackaging drugs in course-of-treatment units and selling them to patients to create a self-financing, revolving fund for pharmaceuticals. The data and experience from this program, along with the rural health survey, led the post-revolutionary government to establish government pharmacies in every hospital and health center for the sale of drugs, the income to be used as a revolving fund for government purchases.

Aside from the drug initiative, the Ministry never seriously tackled the issues of revenue generation in a concerted manner. A few senior officials realized the problem and saw the need, but they were hampered by public statements by higher-level government officials regarding free health services and by lack of personnel trained in financial management.

Cash Flow

The system for cash-flow management was controlled by the Ministry of Finance. Once the annual budget was approved, the Ministry of Finance transferred funds in quarterly payments to its provincial offices. Hospital and health-center clerks prepared monthly time sheets for their personnel and, against these, received advances for salary payments, for which they later returned signed receipts to the Ministry of Finance. In a similar manner, requisitions for purchases of supplies, petrol, or locally available materials were taken by Ministry clerks to the Ministry of Finance. Then, if budget funds were available, a committee of three went to the bazaar to take bids for the items to be purchased. After the lowest bid was approved, the committee returned to the bazaar to make the purchase and then took the receipt back to the Ministry of Finance. In neither the salary nor purchasing transaction did the hospital or health center handle the money independently. The small amount of income from laboratory fees was turned over to the local finance offices. Fees from x-rays were the one exception. When additional film was required, a clerk or technician traveled to Kabul and purchased it from the government's semiautonomous Avicenna Pharmaceutical Institute.

While the cash-flow system was slow and very cumbersome, it did eventually manage to make the money available for its intended use. However, as noted in subsequent paragraphs, the accounting for these expenditures did not provide data useful to the Ministry for planning and analysis.

Budget Control

Once the proposed ordinary (operational) health budget was approved, the Ministry of Finance assumed responsibility for budgetary control. The district and provincial Finance Ministry offices released funds only against approved line items with no flexibility at the local level to transfer funds. The Ministry had the authority centrally to make small (less than 50,000 Afghanis, or approximately $1,250) transfers to funds from one line item to another or from one province to another. Larger budget alterations had to be approved by the Cabinet of Ministers, which for practical purposes eliminated the prospect.

A major difficulty in budget control was the process of expenditure reporting from the Ministry of Finance to the MOPH. The reports were submitted once every 6 months after the last expenditure had occurred in a given 6-month period. The restrictions on budget alterations and the delays in receiving reports from the Finance Ministry resulted in large balances remaining unspent in certain provinces and line items with insufficient funds available in others. This was a particular problem in the personnel item, and this accounted for 76.3 percent of the budgets administered at the provincial levels. During 1975 and 1976, the Ministry of Finance reported that as much as 40 percent of the Ministry's provincial budgets was unspent at the end of the fiscal year. A large proportion of the unspent money was the result of personnel vacancies from retirements, transfers, and unfilled slots. Although there were shortages of funds for facility maintenance, purchase of drugs, and training per diems, reports from the Ministry of Finance were received too late to either make line-item transfers of funds or to adjust budgets for subsequent years.

Financial Data for Planning

Not only were the financial statements received late, they also were aggregated in ways that prevented adjustments for current management or for long-range planning. The statements from the Finance Ministry showed expenditures by budget line items for an *entire* province, submerging the expenditures of each hospital, health center, and other health program. Therefore, neither the provincial health officer nor the central health officials could determine why they were underspending their budgets at the same time that they did not have enough money for adequate program operations.

Because of this situation, the team worked with the Administration Department to establish a financial-analysis directorate within the Department of Administration. Beginning in March of 1978, specially trained clerks were assigned to work in selected provinces to collect expenditure data by program and institution. The personnel had been approved and the training program had been scheduled by the time the new government discontinued the plan following the 1978 coup.

In summary, the major lesson learned from work with the financial system of the Ministry is that small successes *can* be achieved in trying to improve the financial-support system of a single ministry, even when that support system is, in reality, a subsystem of the larger financial system of the entire government. Certain things can be done that will be of help, including the training of personnel responsible for financial planning and management, better records and reporting systems within the Ministry, and the development of the capacity within the ministry to analyze financial data. Occasionally, an entirely new opportunity presents itself, such as the establishment of working funds for drug purchases and reimbursement, and this can be integrated into government procedures and has the potential for a major impact on the financial viability of Ministry programs.

F. Facilities Development and Construction: Necessary, Desirable, Appropriate?
Henry Norman

The initial phase of the project contained no construction or substantial material support. When revised for the second stage, some construction of health centers and training facilities was added. After that point, the Rural Health-Care Project, though funded and administered separately from facilities construction, suffered from the negative fallout resulting from the inability of the Ministry to get the buildings up. The Ministry did not place much importance on the separation between projects and persisted in trying to involve the team in discussions concerning construction—a common and often productive way to attempt to resolve many problems. This annoyed the AID mission, particularly the engineering office, who insisted that the team have no part of it.

There was never any real enthusiasm at AID for the facilities-construction project and no confidence in the ability of the Ministry to put the buildings up on schedule and within budget. It was said that the facilities component was "the price that had to be paid" to get the government to agree to the Rural Health-Deliver Program, an enthusiastic beginning that typified the construction program throughout its history.

Doubts about Ministry capacity to build the centers fueled a self-fulfilling prophecy as AID sought various ways to control the process through what were essentially negative incentives. The first was the fixed amount reimbursement (FAR) concept. This complicated reimbursement principle was never understood by the Afghans. Simply stated, AID agreed to pay up to 75 percent of the construction costs of the building, but only after they had been certified by AID engineers as conforming to specifications and had a full staff assigned. This process was made even tighter by a schedule establishing percentages of construction that had to be completed by certain dates.

The Ministry construction department did not construct buildings itself. Its function was to design the structures, draw up specifications, award contracts to private contractors, and conduct inspections. In practice it usually repeated existing designs, and the specifications were pretty normal. Contractors bid on contracts without even calculating costs, since the Ministry set the price except where a national contractor (one of three or four major certified firms) was involved. The builder would cut corners on the building to make a profit, and if funds ran out before he was finished, he would simply abandon the job. Many unfinished structures throughout Afghanistan are testimony to this practice. Ministry personnel knew of all this, but even if they had been inclined to crack down on inspections, they lacked vehicles and the money to pay per diems for field trips.

The situation ultimately resulted in everyone being victimized. The Ministry asked for a stretch-out of the construction schedule as soon as the agreement had been signed. The inability of the Ministry construction unit to get to the field to do inspections resulted in the AID engineering office performing them and adhering to the specifications that AID had originally imposed in the design. This delayed construction, and as intermediate target dates were missed, it was assumed completion dates also would be missed—everyone blamed everyone else.

This facilities-construction project was a comedy of errors from its inception and should not perhaps be used as a measure of the place of facilities development and construction in general. Properly planned and implemented, it could have been an important positive element in the effort. However, before taking on such a project, all the parties must be clear on what parts they play in the overall program. If indeed the buildings became part of the price for the rural health-care delivery and that part was going well, why permit construction delays to poison the atmosphere? Why not be flexible and work out any plan that made sense and would get the buildings up?

The confusion about the purpose of the facilities-construction program was never resolved. Why anyone felt that it was necessary to improve the construction capacity of a Ministry of Public Health that had precious little capacity to deliver quality health care was a question that was never addressed until the new AID proposal for the third phase of the project, which was too late.

The question of whether facilities construction is necessary involves not only professional judgment, but political decisions as well. Before the latter is dismissed, we should remember that until recently the most imposing building in any small U.S. city or rural area was the U.S. Post Office building. In developing countries, clinics and schools are an indication of progress and development can be important to governments trying to demonstrate this to the people.

The location of a clinic frequently has less to do with its function than with who the government is trying to impress. Many of the planned center sites were not convenient to the population, but were located where new towns were planned or where the local leader insisted. The Girishk Regional Training Center was located at a crossroad where there was little transportation or communication. Its location was primarily decided on political grounds.

The building of facilities in rural areas is desirable. If an attractive building goes up to house an activity, then the activity itself assumes some importance and validity. This feeling is universal, and it can be inane to lecture people in developing countries that they should be doing things in mud huts. This simply reinforces the conviction that they are being treated as second-class people. In general, it can be appropriate for a donor to construct facilities that are part of a medical program. However, it should be obvious that it is inappropriate to do so in the way it was done in Afghanistan.

G. Phases of Systems Development

Management-support systems provide health-services programs with the resources they require: human, material, and financial. The goal in developing systems for support services is to achieve a steady-state level of operation with an adequate quantity and quality of resources for the target systems. *Steady state* implies that the systems have been accepted as routine functions of the parent organization and continue to operate without exceptional outside assistance. Before assessing the team's accomplishments in this regard, a further set of observations from the project may be useful.

Systems development seemed to move through four phases before reaching steady-state operation: determination of need, system design, system start-up and testing, and routinization. *Determination of need* may occur very quickly with simple innovations, or it may take months and even years when complex systems are involved. It involves perception of a problem, analysis of the systemic factors involved, and a commitment by senior officials to seek a solution. This phase may occur between a donor agency and host government before a project and contract are prepared. In other cases, one of the primary jobs of a technical-assistance team is to help the government define the nature of the problem.

System design is often a fairly straightforward technical job and may occur quite rapidly. However, determining and ensuring the compatibility of new and existing systems can be a difficult problem that continues into the start-up phase. The more independently the new system can operate, the smaller will be this problem. Because organizations will already have some type of system for providing resources, frequently there will be resistance to change by personnel working in, and secure in, the existing system. Only strong and active support from the highest levels of the organization can overcome this.

System start-up is the early implementation phase and includes operational evaluation and redesign. This is usually a period of testing technical feasibility and detecting and overcoming the potential points of resistance within the organization and the larger governmental systems of which it may be a part. Advisors and consultants are frequently heavily involved in this phase, but decrease their inputs before the system can move into the routinization process.

Routinization requires the system to go through two or more complete cycles of operation. These cycles might last only a couple of months, as in the case of short training programs, or a full year, as in the case of budgeting systems. In either case, the donor should potentially incorporate some continuing level of advisory inputs into this institutionalization phase. Many, if not most, organizational innovations fail to cross this last hurdle. As the level of consultant inputs is being decreased, unanticipated problems or pockets of resistance may appear for the first time, and system personnel will have to handle the operational problems without the constant assistance of advisors.

Figure 4–1 sketches the general experience of the team in the development of new or improved management systems. The curve is an approximation of what occurs in most systems-development projects, with the time required for each phase determined by a number of factors. Complex systems—manpower development, for example—may take a long time to reach a level of steady-state operations. Relatively simple systems, such as a new warehouse information system may require a relatively short period of time. Completely new systems often seemed to go through the start-up and routinization phases more quickly than do innovations in existing systems,

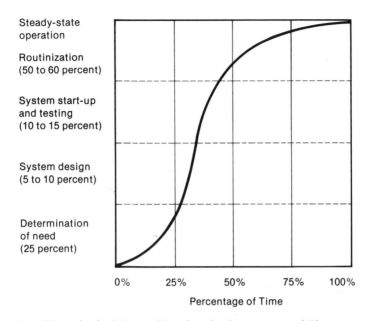

Figure 4-1. Hypothetical Curve Showing the Percentage of Time
Required for Each Phase of Systems Development

perhaps because one does not encounter the resistance of personnel whose work habits must be changed.

Figure 4-2 shows how five support systems developed over time in Afghanistan. The curves are approximations, but in all cases, key events were used in making the judgments. Perhaps the most arbitrary decisions related to the placement of the end of the curves as of June 1979. However, using progress toward steady-state operations as the criteria, the end points used appear to be descriptive of the situation at the time the team left Afghanistan.

The development of a warehouse information and record system proceeded relatively rapidly from the moment the team arrived. Certain portions of the originally designed system are operating better than others, but overall, the system has become routinized. If it were not for the frequent changes in personnel in the central warehouse, the system might already have achieved steady-state operations.

The Basic Health Center Mobile-Team Training Program also developed rapidly through the first three phases. It was at the point of becoming a relatively routine operation in late 1976. Unfortunately for BHS and the

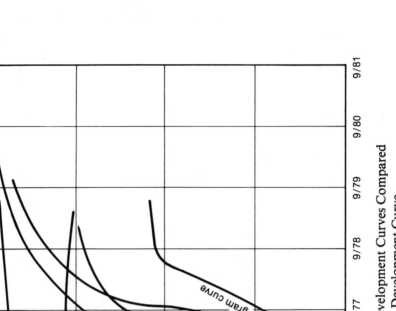
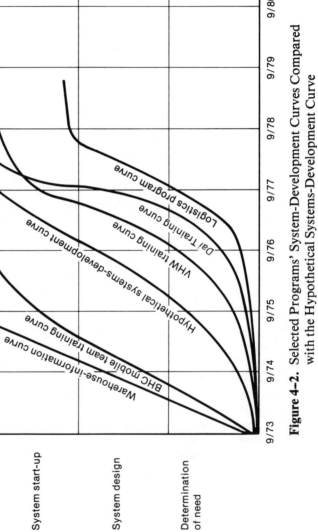

Figure 4–2. Selected Programs' System-Development Curves Compared with the Hypothetical Systems-Development Curve

mobile teams, at that time the Ministry and the team shifted attention toward the newly developing Alternative Health-Delivery Programs and the opening of the first of four planned regional training centers. Up to that time, the team had performed many of the support functions for the mobile teams, and the Ministry had not yet assumed full responsibility. Without close supervision and assistance in curriculum development and in scheduling, the work of the teams began to decline.

Before looking at the other programs, it should be pointed out that the warehouse information system was a relatively simple system that operated almost completely within the boundaries of the warehouse building. Once designed and accepted by the Ministry, it quickly became the routine system used. It was compatible with the general governmental warehousing procedures and was installed in conjunction with the opening of a new central warehouse building. The Mobile-Team Training Program was accepted quickly because there appeared to be no other alternative training approach that could be initiated as quickly and inexpensively. The model system had been developed during the Parwan-Kapisa Pilot Project and, since it was administered from the central offices of the Ministry, was easily implemented in other areas. However, the *training tasks* of the teams were *complex,* and they were given, in addition, responsibility for supervision. Routinization was therefore a more difficult process than that experienced with the warehouse information system.

The curves for the VHW Training Program and the *Dai* Training Program correspond closely with the hypothetical curve. Although the VHW training program was operating smoothly by mid-1977, it was still an experimental or pilot program and continued to have significant team inputs. The standardized curriculum was completed in early 1978, and it is likely that the program would have become a routinely functioning system in 1979 if the new government had not decided to suspend it.

The *Dai* Training Program was rapidly approaching steady-state operations by the time the team left Afghanistan in mid-1979. However, part of its successful installation was due to a highly qualified Afghan advisor provided by the United Nations Fund for Population Activities (UNFPA). She worked within the Ministry with the *Dai* Program director and performed many program-management functions. Should her advisory assistance be discontinued immediately, it is highly likely that program operations would experience some difficulties.

The final support system shown is the integrated logistics program initiated through the 7-year development plan in March of 1977. The central logistics office was opened in December of 1977, and the logistics operations manual was completed in July of 1978. However, the new government replaced the head of the Department of Administration, reorganizing the Ministry; consequently, the integrated logistics program was not completed.

Other systems-development efforts are not noted in figure 4–2. The manpower-development system was still in the determination-of-need phase. The financial reporting and analysis support system was just beginning the system-design phase. It is likely, based on experience in the other support systems, that the development of the manpower-development support system would have been a long process, perhaps requiring 2 to 3 years for the system design and system start-up phases and another 3 years for the routinization phase. The financial reporting and analysis system was a much simpler system and could probably have been designed, started, and well into the routinization phase within 2 to 3 years.

In conclusion, in countries such as Afghanistan, where there is a critical shortage of trained administrators and managers, new support-systems development and improvement of existing systems may be expected to require from 5 to 10 years from introduction of the concept to a level of steady-state operations.

H. Conclusion

Field programs in rural health often can be made to work somehow if sufficient resources are applied in the experimental and demonstration phases. They tend to bog down when attempts are made to implement them widely, even if realistic levels of resources are employed, owing to bureaucracy and red tape, the terms by which management-support systems are commonly known.

To minimize the risk that well-intentioned national health service programs will fail when they reach the implementation phase, only two paths have revealed themselves:

1. The design and implementation of programs that rely on the private sector and operate using the market and self-interest as the motivating forces
2. The design and evolution of management-support systems in the public sector

In Afghanistan, these paths have proven compatible for rural health, and both are employed. The lesson of this project is that the latter—the evolution of public-sector support systems—is time-consuming, often undervalued and underplanned for by donors and host, and essential if there is to be any hope of sustained program impact on rural needs.

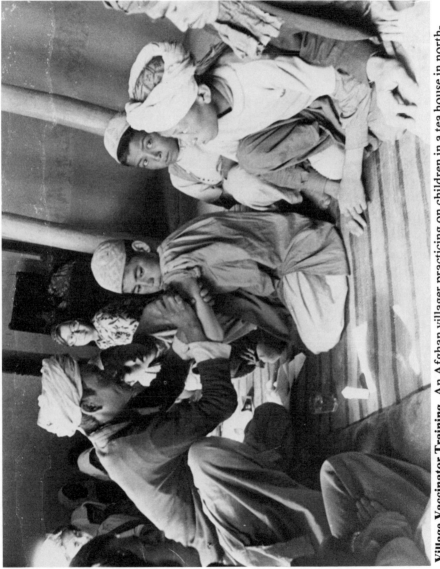

Village Vaccinator Training. An Afghan villager practicing on children in a tea house in north-central Afghanistan.

5

Relationships and Roles in Providing Health-System Assistance

Steven L. Solter

A. Host-Country/Donor Relationships

What Worked, What Did Not

Donors interested the Afghans because they had money, a great deal of money. On numerous informal occasions, Afghans indicated to team members that foreigners were not generally appreciated (from USAID, UN, or anywhere else), but were put up with as the price to be paid to get the money they so desperately wanted and needed. A fundamental tenet of AID's philosophy in Afghanistan (and worldwide) was that among those development priorities shared by both USAID and the Afghan government, certain areas for development assistance should be mutually chosen and implemented.

Unfortunately, in Afghanistan at least, the health priorities of most donors and those of the Ministry during 1975–1978 were quite different. For AID and UNICEF, the important priorities were similar: the delivery of effective health services to those most in need (especially mothers and their children under five living in villages far from a BHC or hospital), the effective management and administration of the Afghan health system, the easy availability of contraceptives to all desiring such services, and the training of female health workers for BHCs and villages. For the Ministry, these were fine objectives, but the important priorities included construction of new hospitals and health centers, development and upgrading of national Kabul-based institutions such as the Public Health and TB Institutes, and international training experience for high-level Ministry personnel. AID was confronted with a dilemma—there were few real areas of overlap between its priorities and those of the Afghan government, despite the obvious need for development assistance given the extremely high levels of preventable mortality in the rural areas. A compromise was reached in which AID would help construct new BHCs if the Ministry was willing to improve the management of their existing BHCs and experiment with alternative health delivery systems for rural areas of the country.

The Ministry agreed, thereby accepting AID's priorities as the price to be paid for the new BHCs. AID was hoping that the Ministry, once

113

embarked upon alternative methods of health delivery and new management systems, would become convinced that these were useful and important innovations that should be continued with Ministry funds.

The compromise strategy basically worked. AID-supported technical assistance was instrumental in starting the *Dai* and VHW Programs and in supporting management improvement in the Ministry, for example. The *Dai* Program has been expanded and is still supported by the government, while the VHW Program has been suspended by the new government for political rather than technical reasons. However, the construction of BHCs has progressed less well. The FAR (fixed amount of reimbursement) method has not worked very well from the Afghan point of view. One problem is that any money that is reimbursed goes to the Ministry of Finance rather than to the Ministry of Health. Afghan officials felt that the money would not necessarily be returned to the MOPH and they would obtain little benefit from it. Also, in comparison with other donors in Kabul, AID was perceived by Ministry officials as requiring an excessive number of meetings and amounts of time in order to reach an agreement regarding a new project. The rationale behind AID procedures was never clear; the complex relations between AID/Kabul and Washington were usually seen as excuses for some other unstated reason for delay. The differences were dramatic; UNICEF and UNFPA were able to move much more quickly than AID to help implement projects (such as the *Dai* Program, which AID basically initiated but was unable to follow up in a timely manner).

Ministry Receptivity to Donor Coordination

The major donors in primary health care and preventive medicine in Afghanistan (USAID, WHO, UNICEF, UNFPA, the Japanese government, CARE–Medico, IAM, the Save the Children Fund, the Indian government, and the German government) actively sought to coordinate their activities. This is always a difficult goal, since each agency has its own separate political and technical imperatives as well as the need to justify itself to its own national or international constituency.

The team was in a unique position to help coordinate donor assistance in the primary health-care/preventive-medicine area. The reason for this was the fact that team members worked directly in the Ministry with their counterparts. The team was generally perceived by the Ministry as *their* team and *their* colleagues. Of all the agencies working in public health, only the team was able to develop a clear idea of what the Ministry's priorities and needs were, since only the team was working directly in the Central Ministry. Moreover, since very few Ministry officials had had much experience in writing project proposals (in English) or even in working directly with donors, the team was frequently used by the Ministry to assist in deciding how projects should be shaped and which should be funded by which donor. These requests were made with increasing frequency after the team had been working in Afghanistan for enough time to allow Ministry officials to develop trust in the team's judgment and their *primary loyalty to the Ministry* rather than to any donor.

The team therefore found itself in a complicated situation. Donors, with millions of dollars to spend, considered Afghanistan to be a high-priority recipient country owing to its great poverty and frequently approached the Ministry about possible projects. The Ministry, being unfamiliar with the complexities of dealing with donors, often utilized the team (or, as often happened, the donors came first to the team before even talking directly with the Ministry) in dealing with them.

The team would then try to mesh the donor's needs, interests, and priorities with Ministry needs and priorities. In many cases, the Ministry proposal to the donor would be written by the team in consultation with Ministry officials. In the long run, of course, the Ministry would have to take over the handling of all relations with donors. The situation as described here evolved during 1974–1978; in April of 1978, the new government quickly changed all this, and Soviet advisors began to play a prominent role in the government, including the Ministry of Health.

This relationship was perhaps unusual, but highly productive. It was possible only because of the mutual *trust* developed between successive Ministry leaders and the management team. The Ministry remained in control and used the team very effectively to serve the Ministry. The team served Ministry management well (sometimes at the necessary price of team/donor relations) and was in turn rewarded with confidence and latitude of operation.

Donor Collaboration and Complementary Project Elements

There were many examples (during 1974–1978) of donor collaboration regarding health projects in Afghanistan. The *Dai* Program utilized technical assistance from AID, commodity support from UNICEF, and overall project funding (including vehicles and per diem) from UNFPA. The VHW Program used AID technical assistance through the team together with UNICEF commodity support, per diems, and vehicles. WHO and UNICEF collaborated very closely with WHO on the Expanded Program of Immunization (EPI). The Japanese government worked very closely with WHO on the tuberculosis program. Even the World Bank's exploratory missions were very much in the spirit of collaboration. The list of such examples is quite long, and the donor representatives of the period deserve recognition for their open and quite supportive mutual collaboration.

B. Host-Country/Contractor Relationships

Regular Access to Decision Makers

From the moment of arrival in Afghanistan, it was apparent that the team's impact could largely depend on access to Ministry decision makers. During the team's service, from 1973 to 1979, there were three governments and four different Ministers of Health, and a separate relationship had to be established with each. Up until the revolution of April 1978, the team via the chief of party maintained regular contact with top Ministry officials, including the Minister. This was possible for a number of reasons.

Proximity and Trust: Team members had their offices right in the Ministry building, often sharing office space with their Afghan counterparts and working with Ministry officials as colleagues on a daily basis. Since the most important ingredient in the success of any collaborative program with Afghans is mutual trust, frequent daily contact was crucial for an atmosphere of trust and cooperative endeavor to be developed. Personal relationships were as important as repeated demonstrations of competence and integrity. Only by a combination of personal contact and demonstrated competence could the team hope to be able to exert significant influence in the Ministry.

Willingness to Work: Despite the fact that the team had clear-cut, limited contractual obligations to fulfill, team members quickly responded to Ministry requests for assistance, even when such requests fell outside the contractual mandate. These requests could range from speech-writing assistance to a crash plan-writing exercises. Although this meant that a substantial percentage of team members' time was spent on activities beyond contractual requirements, it was an invaluable means of demonstrating that the team's primary commitment was to help the Afghans run the Ministry better and to do staff support work when the situation demanded it.

Flexibility of Response: When the Minister approached the team with a particular problem, the team would attempt to act quickly and positively without bureaucratic delay. This was particularly important in such programs as the Basic Health Centers, *Dais,* and VHWs, where innovation had not yet been accompanied by revised procedures. For example, in the testing stages, if one of the BHC training-team vehicles needed petrol and the Ministry's approval procedure would take 1 week for all the proper signatures to be collected, the team could immediately pay for the necessary petrol to keep the training team moving.

After the April 1978 revolution, however, there was an immediate and dramatic loss of access to the decision process. The new Minister and his Deputy were not interested in using the team, having instead, a new group of Soviet health-planning advisors to consult on matters of health policy. Neither the Minister nor the Deputy Minister had had any training or experience in public health, preventive medicine, or rural health. As a result, the new health policies of the government turned to reflect Soviet experience, such as in the training of *feldshers,* or assistant physicians, instead of village health workers. The team chief of party was not able to see the Minister or Deputy Minister, their new counterparts, or the President of Administration.

While different team chiefs of party employed their own styles in dealing with senior Ministry officials, experience with three different Ministers under two governments confirmed the importance of regular communication with, and ready access to, the decision makers. Effective use of the team by the Ministry and pursuit of ambitious rural health-development goals both required and justified the investment of time by the Ministry and the team.

Positioning within the Ministry Operating Structure

An important determinant of team effectiveness was the manner in which counterparts were selected for team members. In the early years, counterparts were occasionally assigned, perhaps inadvertently, in an offhand manner. Unless the counterpart by chance was interested in the work at hand, the result was often negative. Conversely, when the Ministry assigned counterparts who were motivated by the opportunity to innovate, participate in field work, and transfer their experiences to the Ministry's store of management competence, the results were generally positive.

While the project impact relies on improved systems for progress in rural health development, individuals can make great differences in the speed of project progress, and the importance of close working relationships cannot be overestimated. Too often donor agency and technical-assistance staff work in separate walled compounds rather than directly with the people and organizations they are trying to assist.

C. Donor/Contractor Relationships
Ronald W. O'Connor

"When they were good, they were very, very good, and when they were bad, ..." With rare exceptions, donor/contractor relations were excellent throughout the project period and contributed substantially to project success. While the primary interaction and responsibility was with AID, the nature of the project involved several donors—UNICEF, UNFPA, and the World Bank—in significant and continuing relationships. Some attributes of these relations are discussed in the following subsections.

Independence versus Control

One of the most productive features of the relationship was the balance between *independence* and *control*. From the very first, AID, through the project officer and director, gave the team substantial freedom of action. Once it became clear that the team was committed to achieving project outputs and maintaining timetables, AID allowed the team substantial leeway in executing the project. While the workplan remained the basic guideline, AID recognized that, at best, it represented the skeleton upon which the substance of a creative project could be added. Specific examples came in the form of the drug analysis and rural surveys—both were significant opportunities for use of project resources, yet neither were envisioned or budgeted in the initial project plan. In a joint sharing of risk, AID allowed the project to encompass these new work areas at a time when the Ministry needed them, and AID did not insist on a new scope of work or an amendment. For its part, the team took on major additional tasks and stretched the existing budget and resources to meet the opportunity. This flexibility on both sides created an atmosphere of collaboration and mutual trust that lasted more than 4 years before being shaken severely.

Donor Response Time and Self-Interest

Under circumstances in which for 5 years the team was trusted by the Ministry as colleagues and servants of Ministry goals rather than those of any third party, the atmosphere was ripe for innovative development and rapid implementation of new projects. Often this would occur out of phase with AID funding cycles, and in the cases of Basic Health Services drug-supply development, the Village Health Worker Program, and *Dai* Training Program, collaborative programs with UNICEF and UNFPA were worked out. Each donor played an essential role in the overall evolution of rural health services. None attempted to take over or "corner the market" on rural health. The leaders of AID and UNICEF deserve particular credit in the first years of the project; up to the end, they were making appropriate decisions that were not always easy to justify to headquarters offices that occasionally appeared to be interested in taking over all the action.

Local Knowledge: Donors versus Contract Technicians

To the extent that technical assistance is increasingly contracted out to third-party organizations, donors can find themselves faced with frustrating and contradictory mandates. Certainly, this can be true for AID in small-country situations, and it led to the single instance in this project where donor/contractor relations deteriorated in any material way. In a long-term project, contractor personnel may become the major repository of local knowledge and experience in the expatriate community. (By the last year of this project, for example, there were no representatives of the donor community or, for that matter, the Ministry who had remained in their positions of responsibility in country for as long as members of the project team.) It is natural and, we believe, responsible for experienced contract technicians to be considered by donors for project-evaluation and design tasks. If they have substantial local knowledge and are well accepted locally, they have entree that outside "objective" technicians could not be expected to acquire in the short time periods within which assessment or design tasks are often constrained.

Given the short lead times that planning cycles occasionally force donors into, and given the local political realities that make "outsider" acceptance in a small Ministry difficult, AID/Kabul elected to involve team members in the design stages of a follow-on project. The initial project had gone well, and both donors and the Ministry were eager to get on with a major national expansion. Circumstances conspired to the detriment of all parties in an unfortunate fashion. Team members, encouraged to work with the MOPH on an optimum project for rural health-services expansion on a national scale, invested many man-months of team and top-level Ministry time. The result was a large project, including Ministry staff, budget, and policy decisions, all geared to maintain the momentum through the out-of-phase fiscal cycles of two governments and two international agencies. AID/Washington reviewers arrived with a different perspective, feeling that the follow-on project should not have been designed in the field with contractor involvement. Innuendos of mission irresponsibility and "sell-outs" to a self-serving potential contractor who was probably padding a contract proposal altered the work atmosphere markedly. The results, to no one's credit, were a late and watered-down (not cheaper or more realistic) project proposal; a breakdown in mission-Ministry relations, which had grown on an ever firmer footing over several years; hostility between AID/Kabul and AID/Washington; suspicion of the team by AID/Kabul; and team depression over the months diverted from project work to help an AID planning process that produced mainly discord.

AID regularly uses outside contractors in new project design and rarely prejudices or precludes them from bidding on the project in question. (For example, an objective observer, looking at health contracts recently designed and awarded by the AID/Africa bureau, might reasonably conclude that the correlation between *design* and *executing* contractor was remarkably high.)

The trend toward increasing use of contract technicians for project execution in concert with decreasing use of locally knowledgeable donor professional-program-management staff will produce serious dysfunctional effects in some small-country situations. For example, AID/Washington technical personnel or outside consultant technicians cannot always take the time to develop sufficient local knowledge to design projects realistically. A more serious constraint is likely to be the limited time that local Ministry decision makers can give to educating and getting to know yet another set of foreign consultants.

Donors can set policy guidelines and retain decision responsibility when circumstances require delegating design tasks; to further limit options will impede the project-development process without gain to any of the parties concerned.

Project Backstop: Donor and Contractor Coordination

Large and complex projects that extend over long periods, such as health projects, must depend, often invisibly, on backstop support. For AID projects, this involves bureau technical staff, desk officers, and the contract office. The contract officer and contract team are often placed at odds over minutiae that drive both parties to the limits of patience, in many cases without necessity, particularly where the contract team is neither used to, nor requires, the care-and-feeding rules in the standard general provisions. There are a number of areas, for example, travel, transport of household effects, local allowances, and so forth, where a contractor knowledgeable of the local situation can propose simple, flat-rate payments that still preserve the intent of congressional mandate, such as with U.S. carrier travel. They can be both easy for the contractor to administer and the contract office to monitor and less expensive for all concerned. They may not result in a love affair with the contract officer, but they will allow the interaction to focus on more productive topics.

D. The Contractor's Role in Technical Assistance

The team's work as an AID contractor in Afghanistan made several important aspects of the contractor's role apparent. These include loyalty, utility to donors, and project length.

Loyalty

A contractor working directly within and for a Ministry must demonstrate loyalty primarily to the Ministry rather than to the agency funding the contractor. Unless Ministry officials are convinced that the contract team is working for them rather than as extensions of the funding agency, trust between Ministry and contractor may be insufficient to allow effective work. The creation of trust and mutual confidence is so crucial for contractor success in a Ministry that nothing can be allowed to interfere with its establishment. Of course, even though the contractor's prime interest is the well-being of the Ministry's operations, it still must scrupulously abide by its contract with the funding agency. This often forces the contractor to straddle the horns of a dilemma. Incompatible and contradictory demands by Ministry and funding agency force the contractor to make painful choices. In Afghanistan, the contract required that no more than 10 percent of team time be spent on non-contract-related activities. The Ministry, however, viewed the team as a resource to be applied as needed, requesting assistance with activities on numerous occasions having nothing to do with the contract.

Utility to Donors

From the donor's point of view, contractors are useful in that they can quickly assemble a team of specialized personnel to work for a limited period of time. The donor agency has no obligation to these personnel after assignments are complete, whereas it would have an obligation to its own direct-hire people. Also, the donor agency, together with the host government, draws up a specific contract which the contractor must fulfill. Of course, the real world is rarely that simple; the contract, no matter how well thought out, can never anticipate the political and personnel changes that inevitably occur in every Ministry and can make the contract as written obsolete. In this situation, the importance of close personal relations with both donor and host-country officials become especially crucial. When there is mutual trust and respect, contracts often can be amended to reflect the new situation.

Project Length

Probably the most difficult single aspect of the contractor's role involves the amount of time required for the job to get done. Construction of a bridge or a road, for example, provides an end point that is relatively clear, and the contractor leaves when the job is finished. However, if the contractor is supposed to help improve a Ministry's management capacity, the job is never-ending. A 20- or 25-year time frame may be needed to make a lasting institutional impact, while donors cannot obtain support themselves or easily budget for such long periods and, in any case, are anxious for some results within the job lifetime of those involved. The contractor may feel quite strongly that not only are 20 years necessary for major impact, but also that only he (contractor X) can do the job for reasons of personal relationships established and organization experience. Donors frequently view such arguments as self-serving. The contractor, however, is convinced that any new contractor hired to complete the job would be doomed to "reinvent the wheel" and remake the same mistakes so painfully made by the original contractor. There is no simple solution to this dilemma.

E. Advisory-Team Composition

Although every project is unique and requires different combinations of people and skills, there are certain critical skills that are of considerable value in attempting to improve rural health systems on a large scale.

In the first phases of a project, skills in management-system analysis and planning are important. One individual should provide continuity and be available to manage the process, perhaps using short-term consultants for specific technical system analysis (which is one of the few good uses for short-term consultants). The long-term advisor must see that each subsystem impinging on the objectives of the project is thoroughly analyzed, to understand how systems relate and to plan interventions at critical points in systems that are receptive to change. For many USAID-assisted projects, this work might be done during the preliminary preproject period.

The management-systems analysis job can be a difficult one. Both medical and public-health systems must be considered, and an understanding of the epidemiology of the nation's rural health problems is necessary. Most advisory teams have a public-health physician who can do the health part of the job. However, the nonmedical management systems also need thorough management analysis, for which few physicians are qualified. If only one advisor is desirable, the nonmedical management systems analyst would provide the most crucial skill, which can be augmented by short-term public-health physician consultation. However, by far the best combination is to have both persons, with the physician being management-oriented and having field experience.

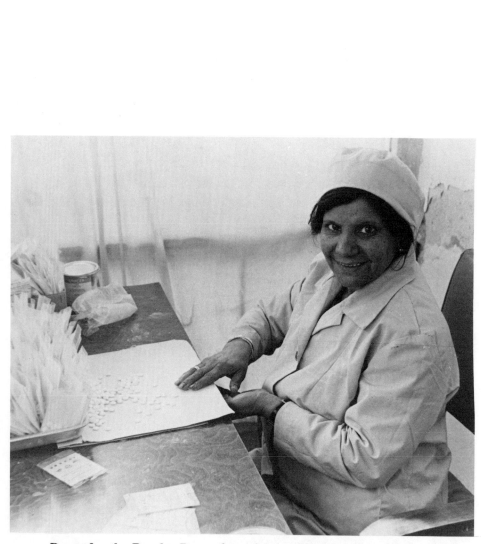

Drugs for the People. Drugs for Afghan village health workers are pre-packaged in plastic bags containing sufficient medicine for complete course of treatment, labeled with instructions in pictorial and written form. This woman is counting UNICEF-supplied tablets which will be sold at a fixed price, generating the revenue to procure additional medicines.

6

Managing and Supporting the Technical-Assistance Effort

A. The Field Perspective
Henry Norman

Management Issues: Planning and Control

Planning was at best an erratic process in the Ministry of Public Health. Huge blocks of time had to be given at a moment's notice to activities that had never appeared on anyone's workplan. Despite the totally unrealistic AID injunction that the team should spend no more than 10 percent of its time on non-project-related activities, far more time than that was required for the project-renewal proposal for AID itself. The Ministrys 7-year plan threatened to take that long to write, and 4 full months of team work was ultimately devoted to that still-born document. In the Ministry, the feeling that "the plan's the thing" was often evidenced, yet once completed, there was little effort expended to carry it out.

The Ministry bureaucracy was very threatened by any implementation scheme for a plan. Reorganization meant new power configurations, and people carefully cultivated allies for protection and advancement. There seemed to be little connection between quality of work and job security or promotion; the important connection was the personal one. In addition, people in high places supplemented their meager incomes through the sale of positions. An assignment to a health center in a populous area meant a doctor could enrich himself in private practice, a situation that was tolerated despite the obvious conflict of interest with his responsibilities in the government health center.

These facts resulted in planning being regarded as an end in itself; the team would help, and donors demanded it. Such a situation created jobs and kept people busy with the unspoken understanding that plans usually would not be carried out. Significantly, the President for Planning within the Ministry had the responsibility for constructing new health centers and hospitals, but otherwise played no role in shaping activities. Where the team proposed or assisted in plans for the expansion of services or training, we were encouraged. However, when substantive administrative reforms were

125

brought up in critical areas such as personnel administration, Ministry officials turned a deaf ear.

In addition to the attitudes just described, there was little understanding of management or the importance and functions of planning. Some progress had been made by the team, but the Ministry's priorities were clearly not in management. (After the revolution, those priorities apparently no longer included even health care. The removal of key personnel without notice and their replacement with inexperienced political operators destroyed continuity and frustrated initiative.)

From the chief of party's perspective, three things appeared central to the apparent success of the program:

1. Location close to Afghan colleagues within the Ministry, allowing development of personal relationships based on shared problems
2. Team ability to make immediate decisions and take action on a broad range of topics, in dramatic contrast to the bureaucracies with which the Ministry had to deal
3. Important team resources—vehicles, backstop, and consulting support—that could be used with considerable discretion on short notice

These are, of course, among the reasons why AID uses contractors instead of doing everything with direct-hire personnel. However, this flexibility and capacity to act decisively and to focus resources on problems must be protected by the contractor and respected by AID. There were occasions in Kabul when AID followed its own agenda and informed the team only after actions had been taken that had a direct impact on the program and could have jeopardized control of the situation. In general, cooperation and communication between the team and the mission were excellent, but the tendency of the bureaucracy to assert control over the program had to be resisted.

Administrative Support Requirements

Arguments can be made on both sides of the question of whether contractors should receive administrative support from the mission. However, removing it in the middle of a program in a place like Afghanistan is not the best way to resolve the question. With a small team, the chief of party has technical-assistance responsibilities, as well as administrative ones. Adding the load of housing, maintenance, and vehicles in a demanding environment requires a focus on nonprogram activities that almost eliminates the possibility of fulfilling the technical role, which is the reason for the project in the first place.

Field Perspective on the Home-Office Relationship

Tension between the home office and the field office is inherent in the development process. Two centers of responsibility are accountable to donors who also have two power centers. All four groups try to deal with host-country authorities, who may not share their priorities and goals or agree with their methods. This tension is inevitable regardless of how successful a program is; indeed success is unlikely without the stimulation of ideas, the necessary refinement of thought, and the discipline of accountability such tension produces at its best. However, when permitted to get out of hand, such tension can be destructive of morale and paralyze a program.

It is usually presumed that good communication can minimize the negative aspects of such tension. Perhaps so, but egos, pride of accomplishment, professional considerations, and personality are very important considerations. They intrude into the communication regardless of the good intentions of the parties.

In many organizations, overseas personnel are frequently newly recruited for the specific position overseas. Their experience with the firm is limited to a short orientation under the AID contract regulations. Once overseas, they develop an intense loyalty to the program itself, but not necessarily to the company. As ethical professionals, they recognize their responsibility to the company, but it is very easy to rationalize a greater loyalty to the program if differences arise with the home office.

The field office enjoys the luxury of concentration on a single program, while the home office is forced by necessity to keep many balls up in the air. The home office must support several programs and do research and development to ensure an uninterrupted flow of new programs. This concern for new projects may appear crass and grasping to the field office, and when it is suggested that perhaps the field team also has a responsibility to help in developing new initiatives, they may consider it beneath them or outside the scope of their employment.

Salary and benefits are also sore spots. The reasonable assumption that one's tenure with an employer overseas will be short frequently results in field-team demands for extended and increased benefits and indifference to the financial needs of the company. The employer who must bid competitively for new contracts, and even for those presently in hand, must keep costs within reasonable limits to remain competitive. Most nongovernmental organizations are unable to offer career opportunities or even guarantee continued employment in international health.

This requires that overseas personnel for nongovernmental organizations be a special breed. They have either a remarkable family situation, make great personal sacrifices, or often have no family life at all. A person is not only required to change countries as frequently as do people in the foreign service and AID, but he must live for much of his entire career with no job security. Changing employers and perhaps living off savings several times is a likely prospect when good new jobs are not readily available. Unless he sets up a retirement plan for himself, he may not be with a single firm long enough to build up equity of any consequence in a company plan.

A development professional in the private sector must expect to deal with financial insecurity, constant change, family separation, and career discontinuity. In the face of these disincentives, the trend seems to be for development agencies to further cut back benefits for overseas employees of private companies. Inflation, tax changes, and other pressures have resulted in the rapid increase in the cost of keeping a professional overseas. It remains to be seen at what point the excitement and challenge of development work will no longer attract qualified people because they are priced out of the market or simply unwilling to endure the instability and dysfunctional aspects of the contracting process.

Meanwhile, back at the home office, invidious comparisons are often made between salaries and benefits for domestic and overseas work. Such perks as houses, furniture, utilities, allowances, R & R, duty-free liquor, and low-cost servants are regarded enviously. The disease, poor health-care facilities, lack of cultural stimulation, frustrations, boredom, poor sanitation, and sometimes physical danger overseas is ignored. Alas, there is really no way to resolve this very human reaction that is experienced even by those who work in both the field office and the home office.

B. The Home-Office Perspective
Ronald W. O'Connor

The Project-Proposal Process

A hustling, aggressive company contacted a senior nurse educator recently regarding an AID health-training project and inquired as to her potential interest in being involved. She indicated interest in learning more about it and was asked to provide an updated biography. Some weeks later, she was called to Washington for what she thought was further job discussion with the company. She arrived half an hour before the team that had been proposed was to appear at AID for the final selection by the government of the country and AID. She was shocked to realize that her name had been proposed as a key member of the team; she did go through with the interview when told her withdrawal at that moment could scuttle the company's chances for the contract. A week later, still unsure as to whether she wanted to go, she learned the company had won the bidding because of the "strength and experience of the team of technicians committed to the project. . . . "

The nature of the international technical-assistance environment in health is that most organizations—both universities and the private sector—act in such a way as to earn the "body shop" title often applied to them. Outsiders are recruited to staff projects, often with little time, interest, or money devoted by the home office to their screening, orientation, and integration into the contractor's organization. They are expected to go to the ends of the earth for extended periods of time and to be backstopped by someone or some group they hardly know and have little loyalty to or interest in—a highly unrealistic proposition. While unmeasurable, the costs of this style of doing development business are undoubtedly high. The symptoms are technician turnover, host-country dissatisfaction, project inertia, and missed contract timetables.

In the long run, contractor-employee relationships must be constructed on a mutually supportive and lasting basis. Contractors have, in large part, only the experience, commitment, and interest of their staff members to trade on; there are few products in this field. Processes, services, experience, integrity, and judgment are the only commodities; all are perishable, and all are transmitted only by people.

The reputable contracting organization's own self-interest requires a high degree of home-office attention and support to technicians in the field. This is difficult to achieve for two reasons. First, field technicians rarely appreciate or comprehend how much is involved in meeting their needs for library research, consultant selection and briefing, data analysis, files and communications maintenance, rectifying charge-account balances, mortgage payments, leave plans, continuing-education schedules, participant training, and getting a clutch plate through customs for a 1973 Chevrolet. Second, donors and contract officers rarely see the value in paying for it. The project is in the field, the home office is just overhead.

Home-office backstopping is equally important in long projects for continuity of commitment. Technicians rarely remain in one field project over the course of its life. They get promoted, transferred, sick, burned out, bored, married, and tired. They move on, as do government and donor staff. In expanded projects, personnel may turn over several times in the normal course of events. To avoid repeating history, one important means of preserving project memory and direction is home-office direction and project backstopping.

Another important aspect of home-office support is legal and contractual. Substantial projects involve commitments between organizations, not individuals. The home office is usually the legally responsible party, not the technicians who represent the organization in the field. They may embody the project to most observers in the field, but unless they are committed for the duration, they do not bear final responsibility for the product. The home office also keeps the donor headquarters informed, a two-edged process that can be pure public relations pap or one of some substance.

Observation of this process with AID can be disconcerting, given what often appears to be an almost complete lack of institutional memory. Mediocre projects touted over and over by home-office propagandists can absorb a mantle of achievement that obscures contractor and project performance. Additional projects are then awarded in part on the basis of "successful experiences" that no one in the contract-award process is able to document; hearsay and claims of the contractor fill the void.

C. In-Country Project Administration
Lorna Hoge Taraki

Introduction

Often unseen and unappreciated except when things go wrong, the local-office staff and organization can be as vital a link for project success as any other factor. Since this project was a relatively complex undertaking, good local-office support was indispensable. It is no exaggeration to state that the entire effort would have been a dramatic failure without it. The administrative assistant for the team notes here some of the significant points relating to personnel, participants, language training, reports, correspondence, commodities, financial information, housing, and vehicles.

An administrative assistant can handle personnel, financial records, and commodities, and she or he can see that the office functions smoothly and efficiently. The ability to work on several different things at once is an asset, since a variety of simultaneous demands and interruptions are often inevitable. Some knowledge of local culture and language is most valuable, but not absolutely essential. For a beginning or small project, an administrative assistant also can serve as secretary. On this project, this was possible for two and half years by having most long reports typed by outsiders on an hourly basis as the need arose. Vehicle dispatching also was part of the administrative assistant's duties until the last year, when a separate housing/vehicle manager was hired after AID withdrew all support services. While many administrative details are in accordance with general office procedure anywhere, experience and hindsight suggest that a few are worth mentioning.

Expatriate Personnel

Folders for each team member facilitated management control, providing a focus for forms summarizing team position, dates of contract, arrival at post, R & R, home leave and departure, passport number of self and dependents, and address and telephone number of persons to notify in case of emergency, both local and in the United States.

Leave records (vacation and sick) were kept in each team member's folder, which was designed to show the cumulative balance at all times. The administrative assistant needed to be familiar with regulations regarding annual leave, home leave, and R & R, as set out in the contract. The allowance or nonallowance of compensatory time and overtime should be clearly understood by team members, and a 3- to 5-year calendar reserved for that purpose proved to be a good method for daily recording of leave information, arrivals and departures, and other events for periodic posting to other permanent records. A card-file reminder for expiry dates of passports and residence and exit-reentry visas of team members and dependents was useful.

The administrative assistant also can assist with travel and shipping arrangements, especially for short-term consultants who need to be kept aware of contract general provisions for weight allowances and air carriers. Orientation of new arrivals and consultants can be smoothed by the use of folders containing maps and local information summaries.

Local Personnel

The number and type of support personnel seems to vary more with the intensity of project activity than with the number of team members. For example, there were eight local employees the first year and seventeen the last year, even though the number of team members remained relatively constant at about four aside from consultants. Local positions at the end included one administrative assistant, three English typists, three Farsi typists, one housing and vehicle manager, one property and procurement manager, two translators, one machine operator, two janitor/messengers, and three drivers. In addition, four temporary drivers had been hired. The largest fluctuations occured in the amount of typing generated and in the amount of field travel requiring drivers, both of which were partially met with temporary employees.

Each employee had a personnel contract, with a translation if he did not read English. The one the team used contained all benefits and limitations, which might also have been separated into a local personnel policy statement. Personnel folders, forms, and leave records similar to those of team members also were maintained, and a local employment application form with complete educational and previous employment information was developed. AID and local-government regulations regarding local employees required attention to workmen's compensation, tax withholding, work permits, and severance pay as well.

The office worked relatively well by giving each employee as much responsibility as he was able to handle. Trying to create a spirit of team cooperation among local employees both by encouragement and praise and by the example of the expatriate team was useful. The "we have a big job to get done, let's all pitch in and finish it, regardless of whose job it is" approach produced good results.

When hiring, without exercising any discrimination, an awareness of local cultural prejudices was important; even though you do not share these feelings, you may unwittingly place two employees in a relationship that is uncomfortable or unworkable for them. In supervising local employees, it was wise to be friendly and interested in each one as an individual while still maintaining enough distance to ensure retention of authority. American-style informality in office relationships can be misunderstood and can undermine respect for authority. This seems especially true of lesser-educated employees in positions the local culture considers subservient.

It also may be wise for expatriates to project a feeling that they will take an interest and possibly help if the local employee has serious problems with which he cannot cope, but to avoid getting embroiled in many minor personal problems of other people in a culture that may not be well understood. Misunderstandings about money can be painful. What appears to be an amount too insignificant to even discuss may be the food for an entire family for several days. At other times, prestige and face-saving outrank even quite large amounts of money in a society with different values.

Cultural taboos, such as requiring a woman to go to a place, as part of her job, where women do not normally go in the culture or family restraints on sending a woman on an overnight field trip with a group of men, also can be delicate matters.

Participants and Language Training

The administrative assistant can assist with arrangements (travel, per diems, language training) for participant training and set up a separate file for each participant. In addition to the intensive English-language training often provided for participants, the project also sponsored lower-level English training (after hours) for some of the Ministry personnel whose job performance would be enhanced by improved English. Cassette tapes for English-language study were prepared for use by field teams who had difficulty attending regular classes.

Farsi teachers were provided for team members as well as Farsi cassette tapes. Chosen carefully, the Farsi teacher often can serve as a teacher and advisor on cultural differences. It was easy to incorporate this into language training because the two are closely interrelated.

Cultural orientation was very important to the success of the team. Occasionally, very trivial acts or gestures can offend without intent. Stretching your feet toward a person, remaining "at the head of a room" when someone higher ranking (familial, social, and official; is present, or not standing when a higher-ranking man or woman enters the room whether you are a man or woman are examples from Afghanistan.

It also is helpful to know the appropriate action or response to cultural events such as births, weddings, and funerals. For example, sending flowers in connection with a death would be inappropriate, and wedding gifts are delivered by a social call on the bride and groom a few days after the wedding rather than prior to the wedding.

Reports and Correspondence

Standardization of copies and distribution of correspondence and reports are useful. A separate file of all documents (reports) prepared by the project was kept and numbered with a master list showing date and name of author as well as a distribution list of each report. Protocol and contract regulations for submission of reports to donors also were attached.

Correspondence and reports that are translated may be filed together by subject or maintained in separate files for each language. The project used the latter method successfully, and a chronological file in addition to subject-matter and correspondence files also was used. A filing system established at the beginning of the project provided room for expansion of activities beyond those areas predicted at the beginning of the project. A glance through the final reports of similar projects and some forethought by team members on statistical data that will need to be gathered for reporting purposes later may help establish a functional filing system. For example, this project engaged in short-term training programs in many unrelated areas. Information on types of training, length of program, and number of trainees was filed by subject matter of the training program. When it came time for final reporting, it would have been useful to have all training-program material filed in one place, possibly cross-referenced by subject.

An incoming and outgoing mail record with numbered envelopes for project/home-office correspondence proved very valuable because overseas mail was often delayed for periods up to 6 months, for example, or even lost forever. With a record, copies could be sent when the original was lost, and someone would understand that his letter was not answered because it was never received.

Commodities

Several different sources of commodities were used by AID, local purchasing, U.S. procurement, and UNICEF. Early in the project, AID was able to provide many, but not all, supplies and some equipment. At midproject, this service was curtailed almost completely. Supplies and equipment were procured from the United States with a large annual order purchased and shipped by the home office and frequent, urgent appeals for single items as the need arose. The local bazaar filled the gaps according to what was available. Procurement from the United States was generally less expensive, since customs duty has been paid on bazaar supplies; however, the 4 to 6 months surface and 4 to 6 weeks air shipping times often made resort to the bazaar a necessity. UNICEF procurement also has its own procedures and extended pipeline.

Electrical equipment was kept as simple as possible owing to limited local repair facilities and current fluctuations that can damage equipment. In addition to standard office, audiovisual, and camping equipment for Basic Health Center field training teams, many metal and wooden items could be made to order in the bazaar.

All nonexpendable items were labeled with numbers corresponding to a card record system. All items loaned or turned over to the Ministry were done officially with appropriate signed receipts. Items that were lost or disposed of as unusable were thoroughly documented at the time because those items eventually had to be accounted for.

Expendable supplies needed a running record with an alert system for reordering prior to exhaustion of supplies. Paper for reproduction or reports was, of course, the largest-volume expendable item.

All commodities, including household furnishings and vehicles originally acquired from AID, were turned over to the Ministry at the completion of the project. This was done by the preparation of various lists, and they were signed by Ministry officials upon receipt and inventory of the commodities. A record of the cost of each commodity was maintained because all items had to be valued on the lists for official turnover to the Ministry. Some furnishings and equipment that did not appear appropriate for Ministry use was auctioned, and the Ministry was given money in lieu of commodities.

Financial

The project maintained both a dollar account and a trust-fund Afghani account in Kabul. The dollar account, based on a dollar checking account in the United States, was replenished with deposits made by the home office. Checks and vouchers prepared in Kabul were forwarded to the home office, which in turn submitted vouchers to AID/Washington for reimbursement. This account was used for school tuitions, airline tickets, and staff dollar expenses. Dollar checks were also written for afghanis to be deposited locally and used for local expenditures that were not allowable under the trust-fund budget, such as language training for team members.

The trust-fund account operated as a revolving advance received by afghani checks from the U.S. Embassy in Paris. A separate local afghani bank account was maintained for the trust funds, with checks being written for petty-cash expenditures as needed. The petty-cash fund was originally set up as a revolving fund, but when a large payroll and sums of per diem money had to be paid out in cash, this was no longer practical, since keeping large sums of cash in the office was thought unwise. It was essential for the administrative assistant to use foresight in keeping the cash flow running smoothly; to have the money available in different accounts at the time it was necessary. The bookkeeping system set up at the beginning was as simple as possible, but room was left for expansion to a more complex level of expenditure as the project expanded.

Per diems and per diem advances for several simultaneous programs constituted the main expense item that expanded, both monetarily and in bookkeeping complexity. Large sums were outstanding since advances were made for extended trips, and these were vouchered when final payment was made. Advances for vehicle operating expenses in the field also were large.

The situation was further complicated because the team often handled reimbursable expenditures to facilitate prompt action in joint-donor under-takings. Both UNICEF and UNFPA expenditures were involved with the team office functioning on behalf of the donors.

Per diems are best handled with a group of well-designed forms detail-ing projected requests, advances issued, itinerary upon return, and a final voucher accounting for deduction of the advance at the time of final payment. If people are traveling constantly, another method of handling advances is to make one advance at the time of the first trip and leave it outstanding to be deducted from the person's last trip. The disadvantage of this approach is the unpredictability of sudden personnel transfer that may leave no "last trip" from which to deduct the advance. This method requires alertness to the whereabouts of the personnel as well as an accurate bookkeeping system at the beginning and end, even though it eliminates a lot of bookkeeping and cash handling in the middle phase. Tables also can be constructed to facilitate rapid determination of per diems to be paid for any given number of days at a variety of rates per day.

The budget for the dollar account was developed in the home office in consultation with the chief of party, while the trust-fund budget was prepared by the chief of party and administrative assistant and approved by AID/Kabul.

Housing and Vehicles

AID provided housing, maintenance service, vehicles, and gasoline until the last year of the project. At that time, these functions were turned over to the team, which hired a local person to manage them. Once organized by this competent and reliable staff member, this office-management arrangement was highly successful. Maintenance service was more prompt than when it was with AID.

At one earlier point, a team member had handled his housing and maintenance himself. The result was a lot of professional time diverted to plumbing and landlord relations. It can be very difficult for an expatriate to understand the ins and outs of dealing with landlords, utility companies, and maintenance problems in a foreign country; more importantly, if it detracts from professional performance, it is a false economy.

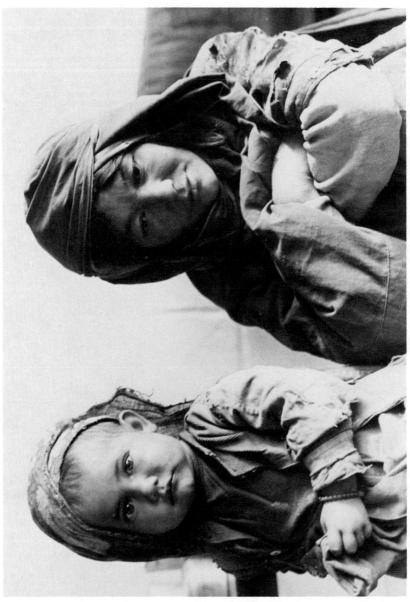

An Afghan Mother and Her Child. One third of Afghan children do not live to their fifth birthday; most of these deaths are preventable by improved nutrition, sanitation, immunization, and access to life-saving measures such as penicillin or oral rehydration.

7

Additional Observations on Rural Health Development

A. The Pilot-Project/Experiment Trap
Steven L. Solter

A health consultant in El Salvador was once heard to exclaim, "We've had enough pilot projects. It's time we stopped reinventing the wheel and got busy helping it to roll!" The frustration expressed in this statement is certainly shared by health workers all over the world. Examples of research-oriented pilot projects that have not been implemented on a large scale come readily to mind. The Narangwal Project in India and the Danfa Project in Ghana have both resulted in a great deal of useful data but, for a variety of reasons, have not expanded to provide primary health care for large population groups. These projects, of course, have been immensely valuable in demonstrating elements of an effective health-care delivery system. Pilot projects have, in fact, provided so much information that additional pilot projects that are not directly part of a national program are often no longer necessary. What must be done is to transfer the rich experience from pilot schemes to the larger scale. The only way this can be done is to do it—that is, to become directly involved with the Ministries of Health in the actual job of delivering primary health care to masses of people, even if it means that research papers are relegated to a very low priority.

The team's experience in Afghanistan may shed some light on the issue of pilot and experimental projects, and table 7-1 summarizes some of their advantages and disadvantages. The Parwan Project, a typical example of a pilot project, except that it was developed at the Minister's insistence as the first phase of the national program, markedly improved the quality and quantity of health services delivered in a single province. Its success could not be replicated on a national scale in Afghanistan without major improvements in the way the Ministry was organized. Numerous observers have pointed out the institutional, social, and financial constraints to large-scale implementation of rural health programs. Many of these constraints were experienced in the effort of the Ministry to apply to twenty-eight provinces what was achieved in the single province of Parwan. For example, small-scale projects are frequently successful because they are managed by universities, voluntary agencies, or local activists loaded with enthusiasm, charisma, money, and commitment. In the Parwan Project, the number of

Table 7-1
Advantages and Limitations of Pilot Projects

Advantages

1. Can be implemented quickly
2. Flexible management structures responsive to project needs
3. Freedom from immediate political reactions owing to low level of visibility
4. Can test technical concepts, for example, training materials, appropriateness of drugs, response of public and so forth
5. Minimizes risks of failure, with relatively small inputs and low visibility
6. Innovations can be tested and adapted and/or dropped easily without disrupting the total system

Limitations

1. Cannot test national support systems, linkages between levels, and infrastructure required for national implementation
2. As exceptions to and deviations from the norm, they can give only limited indication of acceptability and suitability for national implementation
3. May be successful owing to a "Hawthorne effect" as well as the usual enthusiasm, charisma, money, commitment, and flexibility of the project staff and advisors
4. Government may face charges of favoritism for offering "everything to some" rather than "something to everyone"; may ignore political realities
5. Do not test "political will," that is, the willingness and commitment of the government, which is so necessary in the national implementation of programs
6. Very difficult to get government officials, other than the pilot project staff, to take cognizance of the lessons learned

BHCs was small enough that a few dedicated project workers could visit all the BHCs frequently and motivate their staffs to greater effort. When the Parwan Project was expanded to a much larger scale, the BHCs were visited less frequently by supervisory staff who were, on the average, less dedicated than the Parwan Project supervisors. As a result, the levels of performance improved, but never reached the Parwan levels during the national implementation phase. Maintaining the supply of drugs and equipment in Parwan Province was one thing; however, when 120 BHCs needed to be supplied throughout the country, major difficulties in packaging, transport, and getting adequate feedback from the BHCs regarding supplies utilization and needs had to be dealt with by a relatively immature support system. Moreover, the inherent conservatism of bureaucracy was a further constraint in national implementation. For the Parwan model to be successfully adopted nationwide, the Ministry would have had to make significant changes in such areas as personnel and budgetary practices. For example, if BHC personnel were rewarded for competent work and punished for unsatisfactory work (instead of assigning personnel on the basis of political, financial, or personality factors), then the quality of work at the BHC would have been of a much higher order. But to change traditional personnel practices requires a bureaucracy willing to forego the rewards of a patronage/power system of long standing, something very rare indeed. As a result, the motivation of BHC staff achieved in Parwan was not replicated on a national scale.

If pilot projects have severe limitations, this does not mean that full-scale national implementation is easy. The point is that if immense energy and resources are devoted to a pilot project, it is likely that the project will not be replicated regionally or nationally. If, however, those same resources are put into a phased national implementation *from the beginning,* the probability of ultimate success is far greater. Two examples that built on the BHC experience were the *Dai* and Village Health Worker Programs. Conceived from the onset as a national effort, the *Dai* Program's first year was "experimental" in the sense that evaluation and feedback would lead to an improved program. After the first year, the goal was to train as many *dais* as quickly as possible within the limits of the Ministry's training and supervisory resources. The Afghan VHW Program was also planned as a phased national program with 5,000 to 10,000 village workers to be trained by 1985. The lesson would seem to be that it makes better strategic and operational sense for a government or a health ministry to begin a *national* primary health-care program with phased implementation rather than to devote a great deal of time and energy to purely pilot schemes. Pilots also generate suspicion, jealousies, and camps of vested interest more readily than programs that are part of the mainstream. Political positioning is as important as all the technical issues of management support and much more difficult to repair once positions and loyalties are publicly established. Not all national-scale programs will succeed, but the record on pilot projects suggests a worse prognosis.

Despite the advantages of rapid national implementation of primary health care in Afghanistan, USAID elected in July of 1978 to support a 5-year basic health services project that would be limited to a single region with less than 15 percent of the nation's population. AID opposed a more rapid national implementation in fear that it was too risky; officials felt that there were too many uncertainties (particularly regarding the capability of Ministry logistics and supervisory and management systems) to justify a commitment to rapid expansion at that time. They argued that all the major systems should first be tested in a region. Only after this 5-year test should full-scale national implementation begin.

In our view, however, there were several issues to which AID did not give adequate weight. First was that the Ministry was *ready* to commit to a national program and did not want to be limited to a single region. Also, the *Dai* and VHW Programs had been going on for more than 1 year, and the team had had 5 years of experience in the Ministry with Basic Health Services. AID's conservative bias reflected the attitude that it was safer to have a regional rather than a national program; regional success was better than national failure. In the Afghan context, however, a regional program heavily funded by an international donor was looked upon as that donor's project, while that which was going on in the rest of the country was looked upon as the government's own sphere. This is one of the reasons that, in Afghanistan, at least, a "successful" regional project is likely to remain just that—successful, but strictly regional.

In short, *four unrealistic assumptions* are often made about pilot projects:

1. A successful pilot project can be replicated on a national basis.
2. National policies are based on empirical data such as can be learned in experimental pilot projects.
3. If the geographic area of the pilot project is large enough, all systems necessary for national implementation can be tested.
4. The pilot project is testing things the government's policy makers are really interested in.

These assumptions and the experiences led the team to the *following conclusions:*

Pilot projects are safe for donors to support, since they require relatively limited inputs and local government commitment, have high prospects of success, and correspond to the limited budget cycles of the donors.

Local governments may agree to have pilot projects both because the donor says it is that or nothing and because they hope it will lead to greater support in the future. Their real interests are in the national programs.

Seldom are truly new concepts tested in pilot projects. They are closer to "show and tell" demonstrations than they are to experiments. Their most common function is to "sell" a concept, not to test it.

A frequently stated objective for pilot projects is to apply new knowledge under optimum conditions in a limited or controlled environment. However, the variables tested seldom include all aspects of the services and management functions that are the critical constraints. Optimum skill levels are sought or developed in the implementers. Consequently, since the projects represent exceptional situations, the findings seldom can be applied directly to large-scale national programs.

The major factors that determine national success cannot be tested in projects restricted to limited geographic sectors of many countries. These include

Governmental commitment represented by willingness to allocate the necessary manpower, money, and materials

Support systems that deliver the required resources in adequate quantity, quality, and at the appropriate times

Compatibility of the new program with the overall governmental structure and regulations

The ability of the government to introduce new procedures, concepts, or increased activities to existing offices

Compatibility of the new program with the political realities the government faces in needing to provide some services to everyone and to not alienate influential groups with extended programs that appear to spread favor inequitably.

B. The Integration versus Vertical Program Question
Steven L. Solter

Integrated rural development is a phrase that has been spoken and written tens of thousands of times in the past decade, but rarely has been achieved in practice. Once again, a few pilot projects have been able to combine rural programs in limited geographical areas, but integrated programs, at least in the team's experience in Afghanistan during 1973-1979, remain as elusive ideals. The health programs that have had any success in affecting rural Afghans have had mainly vertical training and supervision systems—smallpox eradication, malaria control, *dai* training, VHWs—whether or not the field workers have multiple or integrated tasks. Indeed the BHC itself is an attempt at integration; a theoretical exploration of the BHC is included in appendix D. The *Dai* and VHW Programs were both administratively part of the Basic Health Services Department. However, instead of having *dais* and VHWs function merely as outreach workers for BHCs, the two programs have had their own separate training and supervisory teams, based in Kabul or regional centers. This means that although the two programs are closely integrated into BHC activities, they are supervised by a vertical organization that can exercise much tighter control than would otherwise be possible. If the *Dai* and VHW programs had been totally integrated into the BHCs so no vertical control existed, it is doubtful whether the two programs would have been effective.

The reasons that vertically supported programs in Afghanistan have been more successful than integrated ones are not difficult to elucidate.

Vertical programs can be organized along quasi-military lines, with distinct lines of authority and responsibility at each level. For example, the smallpox eradication program was able to very effectively control its field staff from Kabul and from regional centers. Smallpox workers were assigned very specific and discrete tasks, and evaluation teams constantly visited target areas. Furthermore, vehicles, supplies, and equipment were administered by smallpox staff members without having to have everything cleared by Ministry clerks and storekeepers.

Morale and enthusiasm can be more easily sustained in vertical as opposed to integrated programs. Program promotions and transfers are more likely to be made on the basis of competence rather than on the basis of political or financial considerations. Also, personal supervisory visits from senior staff (which are crucial for morale) can be easily accomplished in a small, tightly organized vertical program, whereas in an integrated program combining a number of different elements, such visits are often far less frequent and are diffused with multiple agendas.

Integrated programs involve combining several existing separate programs into one. Few Afghan health programs are organized and managed well enough to be combined with other, equally ill-managed programs. The result is to weaken each of the programs so that none functions as well as it had previously. To take another example, the Mass Immunization Program was organized vertically, with a number of mobile teams providing specific vaccinations as an extension of the Smallpox Eradication Program. Supervised and supplied by staff in Kabul and regional centers, it was reasonably effective in its mission. The Ministry, as a step toward integration, began to have BHCs take more responsibility for immunizing the target population around the BHC, with mobile teams dealing with more remote areas. Unfortunately, since the BHCs do not have a long experience with drugs and equipment actually in place, vaccines and cold-chain facilities may not consistently reach the BHCs in the future. At least in the short run, the target populations of rural areas in Afghanistan will likely receive fewer vaccinations than they have in the past owing to the uncertainties of BHC performance in this expanded role.

The Malaria Control Program in Afghanistan has been successful largely because of its vertical, semiautonomous organizational structure. It has been able to control malaria within most of the endemic areas of the country. On several occasions, the Ministry has considered integrating the malaria program with Basic Health Services, immunization, or some other rural program. Although such integration should be a goal to aim for, it is not likely to be successful given the existing situation. The BHCs would not be able to handle malaria control on top of everything else they are supposed to be doing now. The immunization program could be combined with malaria control (by either training malaria-control workers in immunization or training immunization workers in malaria control), but the likely result would be a decrease in the effectiveness of both programs.

The Rural Development Department (RDD), a Ministry-level organization, has chosen nine *woleswalis* (districts) scattered throughout the country to be integrated rural development areas (IRDAs). Each of these IRDAs runs a BHC (often with a second BHC managed by the Ministry located only a short distance away). In theory, these BHCs (run by the RDD) are supposed to integrate health care with agricultural, educational, and other RDD programs in the *woleswali*. After 5 years of experience, no such integration has yet taken place. In fact, the IRDAs have multipurpose village workers, called *wolesmals*, who are twelfth grade graduates with 3 months training in rural development (including health, agriculture, education, cooperatives, rural industry, women's programs, and community organization). They are supposed to spend most of their time in villages assisting farmers with advice and providing a link between the village and the *woleswali* center. Observation of *wolesmals* in the field in 1978–1979 suggests that relatively little time is spent giving advice to villagers, and in a sense their fate and frustration are similar to the BHC. Being responsible for so many areas, they are unable to deliver much, if any, practical assistance in any one area. Although the *wolesmals* have some knowledge of health and sanitation, they carry no drugs with them and possess no practical skill that is perceived to be immediately relevant by the villagers. Although the *wolesmal* is supposed to integrate a number of activities at the village level, he has been unable to do so. Integrated development is possible, but first there must be something to integrate.

A central difficulty with integrated programs at the village level in Afghanistan involves the adequate supervision of multipurpose village workers. The VHW was trained only in practical aspects of village health. If he had also been trained, say, in teaching adult literacy and in agriculture extension, the probability of his being effective in all three would be very low. His health work could be supervised by BHC staff, but who would be able to supervise his agricultural and educational activities? In addition, the VHWs were not salaried; if they were required to perform other work without compensation, this would have placed them in an impossible position.

The most important task in village programs is to enable villagers to learn the skills and develop the confidence to try and affect their own destiny. Ambitious or complex programs can overwhelm villagers and destroy their potential for independent, autonomous action. Simple, vertical programs, at least initially, can help villagers control a certain aspect of their environment. With the confidence this creates, other areas of village life can be controlled by the villagers themselves. The goal must be for the project to *work*; the simpler the plan, the more likely this will happen.

The World Food Program Project 599: An Instance of
Inappropriate Integration

Project 599 in Afghanistan provides a textbook example of the problems associated with program integration in a developing country. The primary objective of Project 599 was to provide calorie and protein dietary supplements to pregnant and lactating women and to chronically ill young children. A secondary objective was to provide an incentive for regular MCH clinic attendance at Basic Health Centers.

The project was a wholly integrated one. In the field, the project was implemented by BHC staff. In the Ministry, a small administrative office was established and a junior officer was appointed project manager. A separate Ministry, the Rural Development Department, was responsible for logistics, and the project manager had no administrative authority over either the Central Administrative Unit or the Basic Health Centers.

The Central Administrative Unit was responsible for delivery of supplies to several World Food Program projects, and the transport economies were obvious. On paper, the project promised enormous benefits at minimal cost. In practice, the costs were not so minimal, but the benefits, at least in terms of the project's objectives, were.

In practice, the costs in terms of time devoted to the project by senior Ministry personnel and their counterparts was very high indeed. Because the project manager possessed no authority over either the supply or delivery agents, many issues had to be decided by senior officers, frequently including the Minister. The decision-making ability of these officials is the scarcest and most valuable resource in the Ministry. Much of this ability was squandered on relatively minor problems in Project 599.

While there is little objective data on the benefits of Project 599, the subjective impressions of many national and foreign experts were pessimistic. There is no direct evidence that the food distributed improved the nutritional status of the intended beneficiaries. Much of the food distributed appeared to be consumed by other family members, usually adult males, or made its way into the local market, where it was sold.

Superficially, more progress was made toward inducing food recipients to attend MCH clinics at Basic Health Centers. In fact, there is a clear positive relationship between MCH clinic attendance and Project 599 food distribution. Unfortunately, with the crowds of free food seekers, little health service was delivered. Frequently, clinic staff had time only to sign the food coupon cards, providing no medical service at all. Physical examinations of children were very rare, and for pregnant women, they were practically nonexistent.

The team made several major efforts to improve the implementation of Project 599 with only minor successes. Forms were redesigned, making use easier and saving the Ministry about $20,000 in printing costs and volumentric measures were substituted for scales for the distribution of commodities. The improvements were marginal; of sixteen specific recommendations made to the Ministry in June 1976, only three were implemented, including two in which the management team provided direct operational assistance.

A major project review in July of 1977 brought the Ministry, the UNDP resident representative, the senior staff and consultants together for a problem-solving session to plan for the future. The problems and potential lines of resolution were laid out in exhaustive detail.

Toward the end of the session, the UNDP representative was asked whether he felt that changes were merited. A surprised audience was told— in the face of two hours contrary evidence—that the program was not only a great success, but that UNDP anticipated doubling it in its current form.

On balance, it is clear that both the Afghan government and UNDP seemed caught up in a political process that, whatever their representative's personal views, they could not control. The Afghans were being offered millions of dollars in commodities, UNDP officials succeeded by programming more and more, the UNDP and FAO were pressured to take large grants of foodstuffs from donor countries, and all this led to a severe distortion of rural health services in Afghanistan.

C. Management Consultancy and Local Management Style
James Bates

The design of this project was based on the judgment that expanding and upgrading rural health services required improvement in the Ministry's management and administrative infrastructure. This section considers problems encountered in attempting to introduce new management concepts into a tradition-bound administrative system. Organizational development does not proceed in a vacuum, and consultants daily confront local styles in management that affect and often frustrate efforts to introduce concepts and systems they regard as more efficient and productive.

The Ministry is a highly compartmentalized administrative system, enjoying only limited communication between its numerous departments and offices. Authority is typically delegated either absolutely or not at all. Most communication occurs vertically, up or down the hierarchy, and very little takes place laterally between departments. Decision-making authority centers on a few key administrators, and initiatives and innovations cannot take place without their active support. Accordingly, consultants must spend considerable time soliciting and maintaining this support. This is the point at which different traditions of management first confront each other. The confrontation continues as consultants proceed from initial discussion through research, design, and implementation of their proposals.

Afghan administrators frequently undertake or decline to undertake actions for reasons that may appear to expatriate counterparts as irrational or not based on sound management considerations. Many of these actions may be conveniently termed "local management style." Common examples include the following:

The practice that many key decision makers have of holding seemingly perpetual open houses in their offices. Confidential conversation is often impossible because the room is crowded with people seeking signatures or pressing petitions on all matters of business, personal and official.

The reluctance shown by many administrators to commit themselves to the written word. In requesting or ordering an action, they frequently do so personally, leaving no record of what transpired.

The reluctance of many middle- and lower-level administrators to provide detailed information on the operations of their offices. This often persists even when official authorization to cooperate has been given from above.

The relatively strict division of labor within offices and departments. Coworkers are seldom cross-trained in each other's assignments. When a person who performs an essential task is absent, work frequently stops until he returns.

Cumbersome systems of accountability in property management, which makes quick allocations or transfers of material difficult.

This list might be extended to include many more forms of behavior that appear to inhibit change or impair efficiency. A simple listing, however, provides no insight into why local administrators employ these particular styles of management.

A useful perspective is obtained by trying to understand a specific example from the participant's point of view. A good case in point is logistical support services. From a consultant's point of view, sound logistics management encompasses information gathering and analysis, planning, budgeting, procurement, storage, and transportation. Although these tasks may be divided between several offices and departments, we assume that communication among them is necessary. We attempt to coordinate these tasks to meet such managerial goals as timely delivery or economy of procurement.

The system prevailing in the Ministry is different than that just described. Departments to plan, budget, procure, store, and deliver have been organized, but there is little communication or coordination among them. Department heads tend to refer to their collective supervisor, the President of Administration, for most decisions. They are reticent to communicate directly with one another on problems. For example, supplies for Basic Health Centers are requisitioned through several different channels, with the result that different departments compete for limited transportation resources. The result is slow and inefficient delivery of vital commodities.

While the consultant may perceive nothing but disadvantages in the Ministry's compartmentalized administrative system, it does have advantages to the participants; properly manipulated, such a system gives administrators at various levels certain combinations of security, status, and income. Although Kabul has a modern veneer, many Afghan officials have traditional outlooks on kinship, ethnicity, patron-client relationships, and social rivalries. Furthermore, they are survivors of a difficult selection process, veterans of government service in a politically fluid environment.

A compartmentalized system, one in which communication is limited to a few channels and one in which internal operating procedures of different departments are undocumented, serves as a refuge from scrutiny. If standards of performance are not articulated, then there are no specific indicators for measuring competence or incompetence. The local management style can serve participants by maintaining their position in the hierarchy.

Open-house offices, unwillingness to delegate (or accept) authority, strictly oral communication, complicated accountability procedures, rigid divisions of labor, and reticence to divulge information are not consonant with what consultants regard as sound management goals. They are, however, useful survival tools in an environment of economic scarcity and political uncertainty.

This does not mean that all Ministry decision makers are totally preoccupied with their own survival and have no sense of professional responsibility. On the contrary, many are forward-looking and genuinely concerned about improving health services to the people of Afghanistan. These same administrators often have a realistic appreciation of the constraints in the system, coupled with good ideas on how to get around them. They know that some innovations cannot be routinized without respect for local sensitivities. In trying to effect change or reform, they are likely to use local management style.

Thoughtful consultants working in counterpart situations often can take advantage of local management style to further their proposals. In any case, total administrative reform almost never occurs, and it is unrealistic to plan for development without including elements of the existing administrative infrastructure. Local management style is one of the elements that must be included.

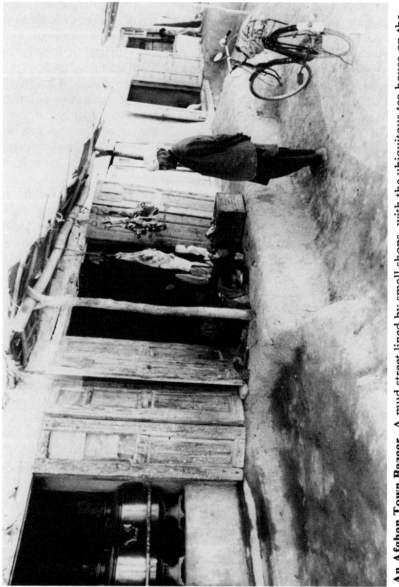

An Afghan Town Bazaar. A mud street lined by small shops, with the ubiquitous tea house on the left announcing its presence with two huge samovars.

8

Implementing a National Rural Health System: Management Experiences from Afghanistan—Project Summary

A. Introduction

This case study describes the experiences, both successful and unsuccessful, of a 6-year effort to assist the Afghan government in managing its rural health system. Working with a succession of regimes and health ministers, an expatriate management team attempted to implement several innovative programs with the Afghan Ministry of Public Health (MOPH). A number of lessons from this experience might be useful to those involved with health programs in other developing countries. Although social and cultural conditions vary significantly between countries, it is remarkable how frequently certain basic questions and problems recur in the effort to develop health services. There must be few developing countries, indeed, in which, for example, the logistics of drug supplies to rural areas are not a major constraint on the delivery of health services. In nearly every developing country, the most important village health problem is felt to be the high mortality rate in children under 5 years of age owing to a combination of malnutrition and infection. Even the causes of infections and malnutrition are similar from country to country: infection because of contaminated drinking water and inadequate disposal of feces leading to diarrhea and dehydration, and malnutrition primarily because of poor breast-feeding and weaning habits.

Foreign technical assistance, in the form of expatriate advisors, definitely has its limits. Using donor resources, almost any program can be made to "go." The difficulty lies in replicability and permanence; unless the Ministry is interested in and committed to a new experimental approach, no matter how successful it seems to be or how thoroughly evaluated, the approach does not become implemented throughout the country. It remains another "successful" pilot project leading to no obvious benefit to the rural poor.

Where expatriate consultants are an appropriate element in technical assistance, their effectiveness is likely to be multiplied if all parties are committed to having them work directly with their Ministry counterparts, sharing office space and day-to-day activities. When advisors are based in their own compound, with occasional forays to the Ministry, there is little chance to directly influence health programs. In Afghanistan and in many other countries, expatriate-consultant impact is directly proportional to the level of trust that has developed between consultant and counterpart; the advisor must demonstrate primary loyalty to the achievement of the Ministry's goals rather than to the aims of the particular donor agency that happens to be funding him. Finally, an advisor's effectiveness depends on his helping achieve concrete results that reflect favorably on his counterparts in the Ministry.

B. Description of the Project

In 1973, the Ministry of Health, concerned about the development of rural health services, reached an agreement with USAID for a program of technical assistance through Management Sciences for Health (MSH) a Boston-based nonprofit foundation. The major purpose of the project was to assist the Afghan Ministry of Public Health in improving the management and organization of its rural health system. At the time the project began, only about 5 percent of the rural population had direct access (within 10 km) to a Basic Health Center. Drugs and supplies were only infrequently delivered. The 80 percent of the population living in small villages depended on indigenous practitioners such as shopkeepers, untrained injectionists, traditional midwives, and *mullahs* for health care. The Minister recognized that the Ministry's capacity to manage the rural health system was rudimentary at best, and he actively sought assistance.

The first three members of the MSH management team arrived to find a highly politicized and factionalized environment following a coup, something no amount of prior planning or detailed project design could have prepared for. Two imperatives presented themselves. One was to demonstrate to Ministry colleagues that the team could help achieve, relatively quickly, some practical, concrete results. The Ministry's prior experience with expatriate consultants had left them skeptical. The second imperative was to develop, over a 6-month period, an analysis of the Ministry's problems and priorities, along with a workplan with specific targets and goals for the management team itself. Credibility depended on achieving some practical results quickly; long-term effectiveness depended on an accurate assessment of Ministry problems and where the team's resources could most efficiently be applied. Two early requests from the Minister focused the team on some concrete tasks: supply logistics and the procurement of drugs, and the Basic Health Center System.

The team was asked to help rationalize the existing system of government drug procurement and importation. It was an example of a concrete, practical request that would turn out to have a significant impact; the Ministry was able to build and organize a new warehouse and logistics system, develop a national drug formulary and pass a generic drug law, thereby reducing the cost of drugs while raising quality and extending availability at the same time.

C. Rural Programs

Earlier government and donor commitments to rural health expansion had focused on the development of Basic Health Centers (BHCs) as the major field unit for service delivery. It was already clear that the BHC development process was slow and cumbersome, particularly in a period of rapidly rising rural expectations. What was not clear was the practical limit of performance of the BHC system given realistic inputs of resources. To determine what the BHCs would contribute, a pilot project was established in Parwan Province using six BHCs from a total of about ninety across the country.

Programs to improve training, supervision, and supply significantly upgraded the quantity and quality of services provided, especially in the areas of maternal and child health, family planning, immunization, and the use of drugs. The initial success of the Parwan Pilot Program resulted in a Ministry decision to rapidly extend the program nationwide. Mobile teams were recruited from Parwan to extend the training and supervisory activities across the country in a politically popular and visible fashion. Without adequate central support systems, the national BHC expansion program experienced reverses that were only to be overcome with the development of a phased plan of operation and regionalization of the support services, particularly supervision, attempted previously from the capital.

In parallel with the BHC pilot work in Parwan, *surveys* were conducted to assess the rural health environment—health problems, avenues to care, and expenditures—with significant results. While the Afghan government was spending about 40 cents per person per year on health, Afghan villagers had spent more than tenfold that amount out of their own pockets. Over one-third of their total health expenses, even in remote villages, were for high-priced drugs. In addition, the survey confirmed the fact that nearly 60 percent of all deaths were of children less than 5 years of age, with diarrhea, pneumonia, and measles as the leading causes of death.

The Parwan survey had several significant repercussions. For one thing, it convinced key Ministry officials that villagers would be able to support the cost of health workers as well as the cost of basic drugs. The survey also helped to focus Ministry attention on rural Afghanistan, where 90 percent of the population lived, but which received a relatively small proportion of the health budget. An extensive follow-up survey, carried out in the three provinces of Ghazni, Helmand, and Baghlan in 1976, confirmed the findings in Parwan and, in addition, demonstrated strong rural interest in having their own village health workers (VHWs). The surveys also revealed the relative lack of interest on the part of most Ministry officials in using survey or field data for decision making. Most officials were either indifferent to the data or used data selectively to justify a decision made on other (usually political) grounds.

By the fall of 1976, the Ministry decided to train village-level health workers. The BHC Pilot Project and rural surveys had confirmed that only a minority would have access to BHCs and that the rural majority were actively interested in, and spending large amounts of their own money on pursuing, alternative sources of health care.

The major international donors all agreed that primary health care was of highest priority, and additional money became available for its implementation. The Ministry, sensitive to the desires of the donor community, agreed to train village health workers on a developmental basis. After extensive debate within the Ministry, it was agreed that 1,500 VHWs should be trained by 1982, under a program with the following features:

> Villages located more than 10 km from the nearest BHC would be eligible for the program (villages located nearer than 10 km already had access to primary care).

> Interested villages would create a village committee, which would in turn choose a literate person (usually male) to be a VHW and would take responsibility for the VHW's performance.

> The chosen VHWs would be trained in an intensive 3-week course at a BHC in the areas of health education, environmental sanitation, personal hygiene, immunization, nutrition, family planning, first aid, and simple curative care. Manuals would be prepared to cover all these topics in a simple, practical way.

> The VHWs would not be salaried; they would be able to sell several important prepackaged generic drugs inexpensively to their fellow villagers and make a small profit. The drugs, provided via UNICEF, would be purchased by the VHWs at the nearest BHC and replenished through a revolving-fund mechanism.

> VHWs would be regularly supervised by the BHC sanitarian; all complicated or serious cases were to be referred to the BHC physician. Continuing-education courses were to be given every 6 months at the BHC.

The VHW Program began in May of 1977. By late 1978, about 140 VHWs had been trained and were working in villages; at that time, plans were expanded to train up to 10,000 VHWs by 1985. When Soviet health advisors came to the Ministry following the revolution of April 1978, the VHW Program was suspended and a *feldsher* (assistant doctor) program was instituted instead, with the team asked to devise the curriculum.

In the spring of 1977, as the VHW Program was beginning, it was clear that a major area of village health had been left uncovered. This was the vital area of maternal and child health, especially the education of mothers in infant feeding practices and prenatal care. Fortunately, most Afghan villages had traditional midwives, known as *dais,* who could be trained to do this job.

With the assistance of the United Nations Fund for Population Activities (UNFPA) and UNICEF, as well as the management team, a major program was begun to train large numbers of *dais* in maternal and child health, family planning, and health education. With a trained *dai* and a VHW working in the same village, the majority of important village health problems would be covered.

By mid-1979, more than 500 *dais* had been trained and were working in villages all over Afghanistan. The Soviet advisors who eliminated the VHWs (possibly because they were very similar to the Chinese "barefoot doctors") did not apparently object to keeping the *Dai* Training Program.

Both trained *dais* and VHWs have been very well accepted by Afghan villagers. The *dais,* nearly all of whom are over forty and illiterate, have demonstrated an ability to upgrade their basic knowledge and skills related to maternal and child health. The VHWs have demonstrated good judgment in the use of drugs (especially two that can be life-saving, penicillin for pneumonia and oral rehydration salts for diarrhea). Although both programs appeared to be successful, detailed evaluation was impossible because of civil war raging in the Afghan countryside. However, available data have highlighted the following lessons from the two projects:

Because of the high level of enthusiasm and support for trained health workers at the village level, recruitment and selection of motivated villagers has not proven to be a difficult task.

Highly specific training curricula with behavioral objectives are necessary for the effective "training of trainers" and for practical outcomes for short, intensive training courses.

Logistical supply and supervision of village workers are far more difficult to organize and manage than are recruitment and training. Incentives (financial and otherwise) need to be carefully built in to the supervisory and supply process.

By allowing villagers and village committees to have final say regarding who their VHW or trained *dai* should be, it is possible to minimize village factional infighting from weakening the effectiveness of the chosen workers and to maintain the focus of responsibility for village workers in the village.

For the village workers themselves, it is difficult to provide incentives so that they will concentrate primarily on health education and preventive activities rather than curative care.

The most important lesson learned from the experience training village-level health workers in Afghanistan is that the idea works—villagers can be effective in relieving the pain and suffering of their fellows—but the political will supporting the idea must be present.

D. Central Management

A major focus of the project from its inception was to help the Ministry develop those central management-support systems which were essential for an effective rural health program. The team and Ministry concentrated with some success on a few key areas—such as financing mechanisms, logistics, and management training—and without success on the personnel system, especially the development of competency or performance-based criteria for job promotion or transfer. The transfer, hiring, and firing of personnel was a major source of power; political, financial, and family considerations were often controlling factors in personnel decisions.

The development of appropriate and feasible *local financing mechanisms* for health care is crucial for those developing countries which have inadequate government resources to pay for all aspects of a national health-care system. When drugs are provided free by the central government, the usual result is that the drugs quickly become unavailable or are sold on the black market. In Afghanistan, it was clear from rural surveys that the great majority of Afghan villagers were paying large amounts of money (6 percent of their per capita income in 1976) for health care, including high-priced brand-name pharmacy drugs. What was necessary was a system for providing effective drugs at low cost to villagers who would pay enough for them that the village health worker distributing the drugs could make a small, fixed profit. This system was successfully implemented by 137 trained village health workers in six provinces in Afghanistan during 1977–1978. Additional prepackaged drugs were brought from the nearest BHC, which was also the source of their continuing education, with the money deposited into a revolving fund that ultimately was used to repurchase additional supplies.

Another example of a successful local financing mechanism occurred in the *Dai* (traditional birth attendant) Program. As indigenous health practitioners in the village, Afghan *dais* have generally received payment (in cash or kind) for their services; after the *dai* training course, the *dais* continued to charge a fee for service rather than becoming paid government employees. In this way, a traditional, locally self-supporting mechanism was continued.

A financial analysis of the Ministry in 1977 pointed out that the budget was being largely spent on urban adult males rather than on rural women and children, who comprise the great majority and who are in greatest need of preventive and curative care. Furthermore, the financial analysis made it unequivocally clear that the number of hospitals and health centers being built would outstrip the availability of trained personnel to staff these facilities and the money required for the high recurrent costs of salaries, supplies, and maintenance. While the Ministry did eliminate plans for a number of high-cost, low-utilization facilities, some donors continued to offer more hospitals. The political pressures on the Minister for urban buildings appreciated by the elite rather than rural programs that benefit the rural and invisible majority were such that rational budget planning was not possible.

Logistics constituted another weak area where the team concentrated considerable effort. A rural health system that runs out of drugs and supplies quickly runs out of patients, since drugs are what villagers are primarily interested in; if they are not available at the health center, there is no perceived need for a visit. Frequent Ministry personnel changes slowed progress considerably; trained warehouse managers would be transferred and replaced by neophytes. Despite these frustrations, the time required to distribute drugs and supplies to all the Basic Health Centers was reduced by 50 percent over a 2-year period; this was only possible because of a great deal of effort and because logistics were perceived by the team as being of the highest priority.

Although many senior officials supported the idea of *management training* for Ministry staff, progress in this area was difficult to achieve. The major problems included "participant trainee" selection based on reward of political services, past or future, rather than on competence, performance, or need; returned trainees without appropriate jobs, which in their absence had been filled; and a kind of cognitive dissonance for health administrators returning to the Ministry work environment and facing pressures to conform to traditional management methods. Without a critical mass of trained colleagues, the institution of new techniques by a few individuals required fortitude and persistence.

E. Conclusion

A 6-year process of assisting the Afghan government in managing its rural health system has demonstrated that the time has come for implementation of national rural health systems that provide accessible health care to the poor majority. Enough has been learned from pilot and experimental health projects around the world to begin phased national programs that can be evaluated and adapted as they expand. Given political support, the crucial element in any national implementation is likely to be the creation of effective and well-managed support systems—for supply, supervision, training, and reward of rural health workers. Given host-government interest and commitment, donor-funded technical-assistance projects can play a positive role in helping build the support systems that will determine the success of rural health-system development.

Appendix A:
A Health Survey of Three Provinces of Afghanistan: A Tool for the Planning of Health Services

A. Introduction

The broad outline of the nature of health problems in rural Afghanistan has been known for some time.[1] Infant and maternal mortality, childhood illness, and infectious diseases have high prevalence in rural areas. The exact nature and cause of these problems, however, have been less well studied and appreciated. How often does a household have an illness requiring some form of treatment? What are the most common diseases and health problems, and which are more frequently associated with death? What are the patterns of illness by age, sex, or location? Which illnesses are perceived as being the most serious by villagers themselves? What are the underlying causes of the problem, including such factors as sanitation, nutrition, child-rearing practices, and lack of basic understanding of the cause and prevention of disease? The health survey of three provinces in Afghanistan was specifically designed to obtain information on the nature of rural health problems in a form that would be useful to the Ministry of Public Health in the planning and management of rural health services.

Likewise, only limited information has been available concerning the resources available to meet the health problems. For instance, the MOPH has long been aware that a disproportionately large percentage of its annual budget has in past years been allocated to support health services that have grown up within the cities. Even a casual analysis of the distribution of health personnel in the country vividly demonstrates the urban rural imbalances. Large segments of the rural population, estimated to be 85 to 90 percent of the total population, are known to be beyond the convenient reach of existing government health services. Considerably less is known, however, about the actual pathways that a villager follows in the event of an illness. Where does he go? How does he decide on the "best" alternative? How much does he pay? How far must he travel? How satisfied is he with the care he receives?

This appendix consists of excerpts from a 1977 study conducted jointly by the Ministry of Public Health and Management Sciences for Health.

In addition, little is known about a villager's attitudes toward the provision of a new type of health service—the village health worker (VHW). Would he be willing to support new programs to make basic health information and services available at the local level, such as the training of a VHW? If so, how should such a person be selected and trained? Would the person have to be paid? By whom? How? One objective of this survey was to gather information on the health resources, both traditional and modern, that are now available to and used by rural people and to determine the feasibility of introducing innovative health programs at the village level.

The method used by the Ministry to obtain the information needed for planning was a direct one, asking the villagers themselves. Persons living in seventeen villages of three different provinces, Ghazni, Helmand, and Baghlan (see figure A-1) were interviewed to obtain information about the health of their household and the steps they take when a member of that household is sick. The findings of this survey are divided into three sections in this appendix: a description of the characteristics of the populations studied, the nature of the health problems confronted in the Afghan village, and the health behavior of rural populations, examining health resources presently used by villagers as well as others with potential for use in a village health scheme.

It must be appreciated that the management process that is carried out after the information has been collected and studied—the linking of known resources to known health needs—is often the most difficult one. It is a step, however, which the Ministry of Public Health has already begun. Over the past 5 years, the Ministry has established more than 100 Basic Health Centers in rural settings. These are designed to provide the necessary infrastructure for rural health initiatives. In addition, the Ministry has designed a Village Health Worker Program, laid the groundwork to obtain village understanding and cooperation, and trained experimental groups of village health workers to deliver primary health care and health education in two pilot districts, Jaghori and Sarobi. Beyond these efforts, other new approaches to reaching remote locations with health services include an experimental program for the training of *dais* (traditional birth attendants) and initial planning for a village drinking-water program to capitalize on villagers' interest in this health problem.

Finally, it should be emphasized that management is a continuing process; last year's answers may not be adequate for this year's problems. A solution that has proven adequate may be made even better. Seldom are solutions final. Thus the manager's need for information is continual. It is hoped that this appendix will demonstrate the role that village surveys can play in providing the needed information and that it will pave the way for additional studies to be used in managerial decision making.

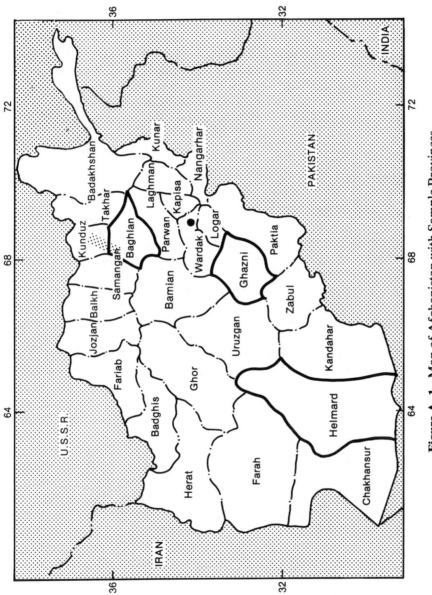

Figure A-1. Map of Afghanistan with Sample Provinces

B. Implications of Survey Findings for Rural Health Programs

Management is described as the process of using existing resources in the most efficient and effective way in order to solve a specific problem. This village health survey was conducted as a means of obtaining the information on health needs and health resources required to carry out the process of managing a rural health program. The most important findings of the survey and their implications for the planning of village-level health programs in Afghanistan are summarized in the following subsections.

Health Problems

1. *Finding:* Infants, young children, and women share a disproportionately large burden of sickness and death in rural Afghanistan; more than one-half of all deaths occur to those under five; women aged 30 to 45 years have a rate of reported illness almost twice as great as men of the same age group.
   Implication: Any village-level health program should give special emphasis to the health problems of children and women. (Such programs might be carried out most effectively in rural Afghanistan through the training of women as health workers.)
2. *Finding:* A relatively small number of illnesses account for the major portion of illness and death in rural Afghanistan; three causes—respitory illnesses, diarrhea/dysentery, and *jinns*—account for over 50 percent of recent deaths and 60 percent of all child deaths.
   Implication: A health worker trained in the prevention and treatment of a few of the most common illnesses could have a large impact on the overall health of a village.
3. *Finding:* With one important exception, namely malnutrition, the health problems perceived by villagers themselves as being "most serious" are those which account for the greatest proportion of illness and death as determined by this survey; 56 percent of respondents named respiratory illness and gastrointestinal illness as the most severe problems they face.
   Implication: Any village health program aimed specifically at the prevention and cure of the most serious health problems should receive a high degree of cooperation and support from villagers. Programs aimed at the very serious problem of improving child nutrition may receive less initial support because malnutrition was not recognized as a severe problem by respondents.

4. *Finding:* Malnutrition is a severe health problem in young children in rural Afghanistan; fewer than 60 percent of children in any age group are classifiable as well-nourished according to arm-circumference measurements; malnourished children had a reported rate of illness almost three times that of well-nourished children.

   Implication: Since malnutrition is an underlying factor in much of the childhood morbidity and mortality, it must be addressed both at the local level, through the development of village-level programs aimed at improving child nutrition, and at the national level, possibly by the establishment of a national nutrition council to further investigate the prevalence of the problem, its causes, and alternative means of combating it.

5. *Finding:* Childrearing practices are one of the contributing factors in childhood malnutrition; eggs, meats, and other high-protein foods are reported as not being introduced into the child's diet until almost two years of age; children with illnesses such as diarrhea are frequently reported as being denied the foods they require.

   Implication: A special priority should be given to the education of mothers in the feeding habits that will be conducive to the health and nutrition of their children.

6. *Finding:* While the actual and desired family size of rural Afghans is extremely large, the vast majority of villagers, 69 percent of males and 91.6 percent of females, are interested in learning about ways to increase the amount of time between births.

   Implication: Given the interaction between birth intervals and the health of children as well as mothers, as well as the expressed desire of villagers for information on spacing their children, it is essential that any program whose objective is to improve health have as a component increased information on family-spacing methods.

7. *Finding:* Environmental conditions in the village also contribute to the prevalence of illness and are perceived by many villagers as being unsatisfactory; 80 percent of male respondents reported a readiness to contribute their labor to work with a government expert to improve village sanitation.

   Implication: Programs to improve the village environment can be expected to receive high levels of community support if adequate technical expertise is made available to increase the chances of project success.

8. *Finding:* Those of lower socioeconomic status tend to have higher prevalence of disease, infant mortality, and fertility.

   Implication: The needs of a specific subsection of a village—the very poor—must be recognized, and programs that will include means of reaching the whole socioeconomic spectrum of the population must be developed.

Rural Health Resources

1. *Finding:* The services currently utilized by rural Afghans are many and varied; in the year prior to the survey, households made an average of 17.5 visits to all sources of treatment, with an average of 3.63 different sources being consulted; both modern and traditional services were used, 60 percent having used a pharmacy, 50 percent a *mullah,* and 25 percent having visited a shrine.
   Implication: There are currently many different sources that a villager can turn to when sick. In designing a village-level health program, it is important to know the alternatives available and to work as cooperatively as possible with those who are already providing important health services to the village.
2. *Finding:* The amount of money now being spent by rural Afghans on health care is by both absolute and relative terms very large; the median annual reported expenditure is 1000 Afghanis (50 Afghanis equal $1); 7.4 percent of the estimated household income is spent on health.
   Implication: Since villagers are already spending large amounts of money for health services, they should be capable of supporting local health programs, such as a village health worker, provided that the programs have a demonstrated value to the village.
3. *Finding:* Medicines represent the single most expensive item in the villagers' health budget; 37.0 percent of the annual health expenditure is spent at the pharmacy, with an average per-visit cost of 248 Afghanis.
   Implication: One of the greatest savings in the cost of health care to villagers could be made by increasing access to low-cost, high-quality medicines through programs carried out in existing pharmacies, BHCs, village shops, or by village health workers.
4. *Finding:* Villagers' satisfaction with the services currently available to them varies; 64.3 percent are satisfied with the BHC, but only 31 percent felt that the *dokhan* was an adequate source of medicines; 33 percent felt that the BHC was the best source of treatment outside of the household for an illness, while only 0.9 percent named the local private doctor. The most frequently mentioned health improvement needed was access to medicines.
   Implication: The respondents report being quite satisfied with the services available through the Basic Health Center, except in its role in distributing medicines. The expressed desire of villagers for increased availability of medicines provides an indication that any program

aimed at improving access to drugs would meet with a high level of village support.

5. *Finding:* Villagers are strongly supportive of the concept of a village health worker; 78 percent of males and 95 percent of females felt that a VHW was feasible for their village. A significant number of individuals were able to name a person, in many cases a woman, who they felt would make a good VHW.

   Implication: Attempts to institute a VHW Program can expect to be favorably received by villagers.

6. *Finding:* Informants agreed that VHWs should be paid, but were divided on how he or she should be paid, 43 percent stating that the village should pay and slightly more stating that the government should pay.

   Implication: More evaluation based on actual experience will be required to determine whether villagers are able to support a health worker and to determine the best means for collecting the money in the village.

7. *Finding:* A relatively large percent (27 percent) of males stated that they would allow their wife or daughter to be trained as a VHW; 34 percent felt that it would be possible to find a woman from the village who would be able to leave the village for some time for training.

   Implication: In most villages it may be possible to recruit and train a woman as a VHW for the crucial role of working with mothers on the improvement of child nutrition and health.

8. *Finding:* Mobility of women is severely limited by the restrictions placed on their travel. However, 44 percent report being able to visit a BHC unescorted by a male. Almost half the women listen to the radio at least once a week.

   Implication: While the channels for the diffusion of information into the Afghan village are currently quite narrow, especially for the women, the potential exists for the use of innovative mass media radio techniques to improve maternal knowledge and childrearing practices. The BHC exists as a legitimate object of travel for many women and can serve as an important educational center as well as a location for women to communicate with one another.

9. *Finding:* The opportunities that a household has for the care of its sick members, as well as its attitudes concerning what is appropriate treatment, are affected by its socioeconomic status. Likewise, opportunities for these households to receive information that would assist them in improving and maintaining their health appear to be more restricted than for wealthier households.

   Implication: Plans for the improvement of village health conditions must take the heterogeneity of the village population into consideration. Specifically, provision must be made to include access for the poor to health services in any program that is designed to make use of available village resources.

Conclusion

No research is useful unless its results are helpful to managers in making decisions that affect their programs. As such, the results of a study or survey must be relevant, understandable, and—of great importance—timely. Table A-1 summarizes some of the immediate applications the findings of this report have had, since the time that a preliminary report was available, for the planning of a Village Health Worker Program.[2] In addition, it presents in summary form some of the implications of the study for future Ministry of Public Health programs aimed at improving rural health. The final test of the usefulness of the survey, however, will be found in whether or not it has served a role in accelerating the rate at which health standards in the Afghan village are improved.

C. Methodology

The provinces selected for the study were determined by the Ministry of Health in accordance with its overall scheme for the expansion of rural health services. Within each of the provinces selected—Ghazni, Helmand, and Baghlan—two established Basic Health Centers (BHCs) were chosen as focal points for village selection. Selection of BHCs was based on length of operation (and thus their potential historical impact on the community), as well as on the desire to achieve a representative variation of geographic, social, and economic conditions within each province. Village selection was accomplished by preparing grid maps of areas adjacent to the selected BHCs and by random selection of villages at 1 km, 10 km, and 15 km from the health center. Within each village, household selection was done systematically, using prelists of households developed by a random start method. Depending on the size of the village, every second or third household on the prelist form was sampled. Within a household, an attempt was made to interview an adult male and an adult female, preferably, but not exclusively, a husband and a wife. Respondents were required to be adult (over 18) and permanent members of the household, with preference being given to heads of households and their spouses. Only one wife was interviewed per polygamous marriage. The discrepancy between the number of female interviews conducted (486) and the number of male interviews (237) primarily reflects the fact that during the interview period—August to October— many men were engaged in agricultural activities at a distance from their village.

Table A-1
Immediate Applications of the Three-Province Survey

Conclusions and Findings Supporting Conclusions		Planning Applications	
Conclusion	Findings Supporting Conclusion	Immediate Applications to VHW Program	Probable/Possible Future Applications

A. The Health Problem

Conclusion	Findings Supporting Conclusion	Immediate Applications to VHW Program	Probable/Possible Future Applications
1. Infants, young children, and women bear disproportionately large share of the burden of sickness and death.	Half of all deaths are under age 5 years; infant mortality rate 157; women aged 30 to 45 have incidence of illness twice men of same age group.	VHW Training Program designed to emphasize problems of children and women. Commitment increased to recruit women whenever possible.	Infant mortality rate and childhood and maternal morbidity rates to be used in evaluation of the impact of village-level health programs.
2. A relatively small number of illnesses, many preventable or treatable at village level, account for major portion of illness and death.	Respiratory illnesses, diarrhea/dysentery, and *jinns* account for 50 percent of all recent deaths and 60 percent of all recalled child deaths.	VHW trained to recognize and treat major health problems; treatment protocols and medical supplies standardized for specific therapy regimens.	Investigation into etiology of *jinns*; development of maternal tetanus immunization program.
3. Health problems perceived by villages as most serious account for majority of illness (except malnutrition and *jinns*, which are not viewed as serious).	Fifty-six percent of respondents named respiratory illness and gastrointestinal problems as "most serious." *Jinns* and malnutrition not mentioned as health problem.	VHW trained in methods of obtaining village cooperation by eliciting felt needs and addressing answers to these; also taught importance of making villagers aware of unrecognized needs.	Role of VHW in village education; the BHC as a source of education for women.
4. Malnutrition is a severe health problem among young children.	Less than 50 percent of children aged 12 to 60 months classifiable as well-nourished.	VHW training organized to stress the role of nutrition in illness and possible means of intervention.	More detailed nutritional survey to further define problem and underlying causes. Formation of a National Nutrition Planning Council.
5. Childrearing practices are major contribution to malnutrition.	Meats, eggs, and high-protein food reputed not to be introduced until 2 years; some children not fed during illnesses.	VHW, especially women, taught food preparation, food values, and methods of working with mothers to improve nutrition.	Radio programs designed to promote nutrition education; BHCs developed as nutrition training center for villages

Table A-1 (continued)

	Conclusions and Findings Supporting Conclusions		Planning Applications	
Conclusion	Findings Supporting Conclusion		Immediate Applications to VHW Program	Probable/Possible Future Applications
6. Although desired family size remains large, men and women are both interested in learning about child-spacing methods.	Sixty-nine percent of men and 91.6 percent of women report being interested in learning about spacing.		VHW curriculum includes section on rationale and methods of family planning; male and female contraceptives included in VHW basic supply kit.	Female VHWs to promote contraception for maternal and child health objective.
7. Environmental conditions in village contribute to illnesses.	Many villagers perceive the sanitation facilities and drinking water supply to be inadequate; 80 percent of men willing to contribute to improvement.		Basics of environmental sanitation taught to VHWs; technical backup provided to VHWs who begin village projects.	Specific environmental health programs of MOPH working directly with villagers.
B. Village Health Resources				
1. Services currently utilized are many and varied, modern and traditional.	Households average 17.5 visits to sources of treatment a year; average of 3.63 different sources; 50 percent of household use pharmacy, BHC, and *mullah* during year.		Selection process for VHWs includes review of those currently providing health services; VHW curriculum includes discussion of total resources available.	Retraining of traditional birth attendants; promotion of shops for sale of medicines.
2. Household health expenditure now very high in relative and absolute terms.	Median reported household health expenditures is 1,000 Afghanis, 7.4 percent of the estimated household income.		VHW program will test feasibility of full village support; various payment schemes will be tried including fee-for-service and profit from sale of drugs.	Charge for services and medications provided at BHCs.
3. Medicines represent single most expensive item in health budget.	Thirty-seven percent of annual health expenditure spent in pharmacy, average of 248 Afghanis per visit.		Basic essential medicines to be provided to VHW at start; resupply through BHC at minimal cost; control over amount that can be charged set by village leaders or by MOPH.	Continued efforts to reduce cost of drugs through improved national purchase and production schemes.

4.	Great variation in villager satisfaction with available services; improvement desirable in many services.	Sixty-four percent satisfied with BHC; only 31 percent with medications available through village shops.	Access to medicine to be one objective of VHW program; BHC referral and supervisory system for VHWs.	Use of shops for medicine distribution; government support for services now considered valuable, such as bonesetter.
5.	Village health worker concept seen as feasible by many.	Seventy-eight percent of men and 95 percent of women felt VHW would be appropriate and feasible in their village.	Current program will evaluate those conditions which contribute to the success of VHW Program.	Results of evaluation to be used in expansion of VHW program.
6.	VHWs will have to be compensated; exact mechanism will depend on characteristic of village.	Eighty percent felt VHWs would have to be paid; 43 percent felt the village should pay; 47 percent felt that the government should support.	Current program to experiment with payment schemes.	Plan future VHW payment in accordance with evaluation of current program.
7.	In most villages it should be possible to recruit and train women as VHWs.	Twenty-seven percent of men would allow their wives or daughters to be VHWs; 34 percent felt it would be possible to find female VHWs in their village.	Background research being done to determine methods of recruiting women and obtaining village understanding of their roles. Six women recruited from first two experimental sites.	Each village to have at least one female VHW.
8.	Mobility and channels of communication for village women are severely limited. BHC is a potential legitimate meeting and education center. Radio has immense potential for diffusion of information.	Fifty percent of women reported listening to radio; only 3 percent of women claimed to be able to visit friends unescorted in their own village; 44 percent reported being able to visit BHC.	Female VHW role designed to emphasize the diffusion of information to village women.	Mass-media education via radio. Use of BHC as center for education and communication.
9.	The socioeconomic status of household influences health standards and behavior.	The annual health expenditure of households ranges from 0 to 5,000 Afghanis. Poorer households have higher rates of illness.	VHW remuneration schemes planned to take into consideration extreme poverty of many households.	Nutrition studies to determine roles of poverty and lack of education in malnutrition.

All interviews were carried out by trained male and female interviewers using separate interview forms for men and women that had been designed, pretested, and revised before the start of the survey. Male and female questionnaires contained both overlapping and different questions. For example, only women were asked questions concerning childrearing behavior, while both men and women supplied information about illnesses, health expenditures, and attitudes toward health services. A team of two female interviewers met with each female, while a single male interviewer was used for the male interview. Each interview required between 40 and 50 minutes to complete, a length that did not appear to affect cooperation, as judged from respondents' compliance. No effort was made to coerce interviewee cooperation. For example, in one of the sample villages originally selected, suspicion and lack of cooperation made it necessary to seek an alternative sample site. Respondents were given no rewards for participation, and care was taken to explain to the village that participation in the survey did not imply a guarantee of any future government help.

Interviewers were trained over a 2-week period and received both classroom instruction, field practice, and performance evaluation. During interviewing, quality-control checks were carried out by the field team supervisor and the training staff. The number of interviews completed during the 3 months of field work is shown in table A–2.

Coding of questionnaires was done by Ministry of Public Health personnel with the supervision of the staff of the management team. Keypunching and data preparation were performed by Afghan Business Machines in Kabul, and data analysis was done in Cambridge, Massachusetts by the staff of Management Sciences for Health, Inc. The use of partially processed questionnaires and the cooperation of all those involved in the data processing made it possible to produce a preliminary report of survey findings within 3 months of completion of the survey, a turn around time that allowed the results of the survey to be used in the planning of the Village Health Worker Program.

Since one goal of the survey was to obtain information on the nutrition and growth of village children, all children aged one to four years in a household were weighed using hanging Salter scales. In addition, each child's height and midarm circumference were determined using standardized measuring instruments.

D. Findings of Survey

Demographic Profile of the Population Sampled

It is often useful to describe the characteristics of a population sampled, including age and sex distribution, the birth rate, the death rate, and the size

Table A-2
Distribution of Interviews, by Province and Village

Province	Village	Female Interviews	Male Interviews	Total Interviews
Ghazni	Khonadai	32	27	59
	Khonsal Kosh	36	11	47
	Jabaar Khel	22	17	39
	Khanadara	21	9	30
	Bakhtyar	30	16	46
Total Ghazni Province		141	80	221
Baghlan	Tawashakh	26	12	38
	Khoja Khede	31	9	40
	Kona Qala	27	16	43
	Qashlak Qala	30	14	44
	Na Bahar	29	14	43
	Ghazmarq	27	10	37
Total Baghlan Province		170	75	245
Helmand	Loye Bagh	31	16	47
	Nawliabad	30	14	44
	Saidabad	31	13	44
	Nowzad	27	10	37
	Konjak	32	11	43
	Kanghai	24	18	42
Total Helmand Province		175	82	257
Survey total		486	237	723

of households. A thorough description of a population makes it possible to compare the findings from surveys carried out at different times or different locations. For example, only if important characteristics of two populations are known to be very similar would it be legitimate to make comparisons of such basic measurements as birth or mortality rates. An analysis of demographic data also helps in identifying and understanding regional differences in population over time.

Additionally, demographic information assists in determining whether the population sampled is genuinely representative of the entire population. As an extreme example, any rural survey that included only *maliks* or large landholders as informants would immediately be suspect as not being representative, and its results would have to be interpreted in light of this potential bias.

Characteristics of the Population: The population surveyed included 3,483 individuals living in 486 households. Of these, 51.2 percent were males. The mean age of household members was 21.0 years, with 49.4 percent of the population below the age of 15 years. Only 3.9 percent were over 65. The dependency ratio of the population—those under 15 years of age or over 65 as a percentage of those 15 to 65 years of age—was 114. A breakdown of the population by age and sex (figure A-2) demonstrates the relative decrease in females over males in the age groups 35 years and over. This differential survival, which has been documented by the national demographic survey as well,[3] may possibly be attributable to the effects of continued childbirth on maternal health. Thirty-eight percent of all household members were married at the time of the survey and 2.5 percent were widowed. Among the 486 female respondents, 23.0 percent reported being a cowife. The mean number of wives per husband was 1.24.

Educational levels and literacy of household members over 15 years of age was as follows:

	Mean Years of School	Percent Having Attended School
Male	1.99	26
Female	0.27	5

Thirty percent of the adult men and 3.5 percent of the adult women were reported as being literate.

The principal reported occupations of males over fifteen were

Farmer	47.2%
No occupation	12.6%
Student	6.3%
Laborer	5.7%
Shopkeeper	4.3%
Mullah	2.8%
Clerk	2.5%
All others	18.6%

The mean age of male respondents to the questionnaire was 46.5 years, while that of female respondents was 35.1 years. Almost 90 percent of men interviewed were heads of households, and 86 percent of the women were wives of heads of households. In 98 percent of the 237 households in which a male was interviewed, a female was also interviewed.

Household Characteristics: As mentioned earlier, there were 3,483 individuals enumerated in the 486 households in the sample, thus an average of 7.17 persons per household. The mean number of rooms per household was 2.25, with the distribution broken down as follows:

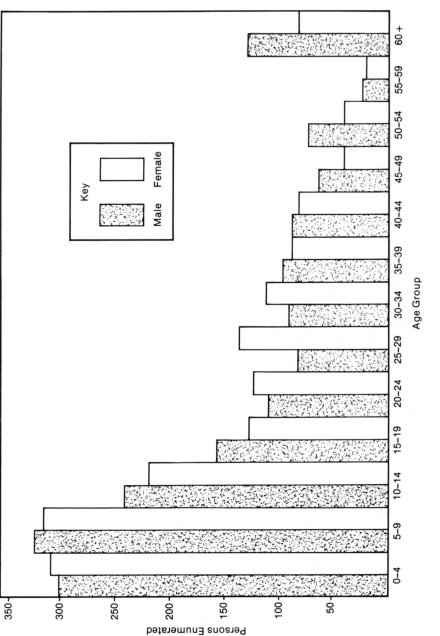

Figure A–2. Age and Sex Profile of Population Studied

Number of Rooms	Percent of Households
1	38.9
2	31.1
3	14.8
4	7.3
5	1.8
6	3.8
7 or more	2.3

The average number of persons per room was 3.18, a figure that indicates extreme crowding.

As described in section A.2, villages were selected at varying distances from Basic Health Centers in order to allow for comparisons in health-seeking behavior. Distribution of villages by distance from the health center is 1 km, 40 percent; 10 km, 35 percent; and 15 km, 25 percent.

A number of previous surveys have demonstrated the difficulty in obtaining reliable information on the economic status of households in Afghanistan. Thus, in this survey, no attempt was made to obtain information on the annual household income. However, owing to the importance of socioeconomic status as a determinant of illness and health behavior, two indicators were used. The first was the number of rooms in a household and the crowding factor, that is, the number of persons per room. The second indicator was a subjective one: Female interviewers were asked at the completion of each interview, "How would you judge the economic standard of this household in relation to others in the village?" The classification is as follows:

Extremely poor	34.7%
Poorer than average	38.6%
Average	20.4%
Above average	4.8%
Extremely wealthy	1.5%

While a disproportionate number of households were rated as being poor by interviewers, the classification system does allow for the division of households into three very nearly equal categories: extremely poor, poorer than average, and average or above. A socioeconomic standard (SES) was determined for each household using a formula that weighs both the crowding factor and the interviewer's evaluation of the household's economic standard. The SES with classifications of very poor, poor, and average or better is the standard that has been used throughout this report to make socioeconomic comparisons.

Fertility, Mortality, and Growth Rates: Female respondents, mean age 35.1 years, had an average of 3.93 living children and 5.82 children ever born. The number of children living and ever born for women in 5-year intervals is, however, a better indicator of overall fertility. These data are presented in figure A-3.

As figure A-3 points out, women of completed reproductive age, that is, over 45, reported having had an average of 9.37 children ever born and 5.67 still living; 40 percent of their offspring were reported to have died. Age-specific fertility rates for all women, and for married women alone are presented in table A-3.

The total fertility rate, considered one of the best single cross-sectional measures of fertility, estimates the average number of children that a woman would bear is 9.23 if she went through her reproductive years exposed to the age-specific fertility rate for the women interviewed—that is, a woman with completed fertility would have an average of 9.23 births if the rates in table A-3 remained unchanged throughout her reproductive years.

The crude birth rate is the number of births per 1,000 total population per year. In the households interviewed, there had been a total of 169 births, or 48.5 births per 1,000 in the period since the previous *Jeshyn* (national day). When this rate is standardized to a single complete year, the crude birth rate is 41.3 per 1,000 total population.

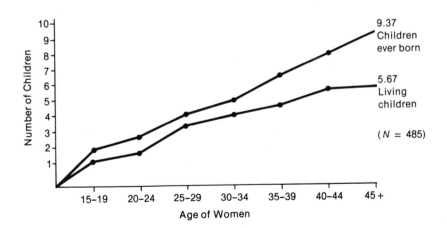

Figure A-3. Living Children and Children Ever Born for Female Respondents, by 5-Year Groups

Table A-3
Age-Specific Fertility Rates for Married Women and All Women

Age Group	Percent of Women Married	Married Women Fertility per 1,000 Women per Year	All Women Fertility per 1,000 Women per Year
15–19	39.1	440	172
20–24	79.5	488	388
25–29	93.4	400	374
30–34	95.5	382	365
35–39	96.6	328	317
40–44	91.5	227	208
45–49	84.6	27	23

The number of deaths in the population during the same recall period was 98, giving a crude death rate of 24.2 per 1,000 after adjustment for a single year. Current vital rates lead to a growth rate of 1.71 percent for the rural villages studied. This would lead to a doubling of the population within 36 years.

The infant mortality rate, or the number of children under 1 year of age who die per 1,000 live births in a year for the population studied, was 157. Almost 60 percent of all deaths in the preceding year were of children under 5 years of age, with the breakdown by single-year intervals as follows:

Age of Death (N = 59)	Percent of All Deaths 0–5 Years
0–1	43.2
1–2	29.3
2–3	15.5
3–4	3.4
4–5	8.6

While the three-province survey was not designed as a demographic study, some comparison of its demographic findings with other surveys carried out in Afghanistan is noteworthy, as is a comparison of the vital data of rural Afghanistan with selected other countries. These comparisons are presented in tables A–4 and A–5, respectively.

Rural Health Problems and Needs

Any attempt to improve health services should be planned with as thorough an understanding of the nature and causes of the specific health problems as

Table A-4

A Comparison of Population Characteristics from the Three-Province Survey with Other Afghan Surveys

Parameter	Three-Province Survey	National Demographic Survey	WHO/Infant Mortality Survey	Buck et al. Four-Village Survey	CINAM Survey	Parwan-Kapisa Survey
Infant mortality rate	157	185	183	205	154	150–200
Crude birth rate	41.3	43.0	45.6	44.6	44.0	43.0
Crude death rate	24.2	21.0	—	—	20.0	20.0
Growth rate	1.7%	2.2%	—	—	2.4	2.3
Maternal mortality rate	—	64.2 per 100,000	—	—	—	—
Women age 45, number children ever born	9.3	7.7	—	—	—	7.7[a]
Women, age 45, number children died	3.6	3.4	—	—	—	2.6[a]
Persons per household	7.2	6.2	—	—	7.4	6.2

[a] Ages 35 to 39.

Table A-5

Comparison of Population Characteristics of Afghanistan with Those of Neighboring Countries

	Afghanistan	Nepal	India	Iran	Iraq	Pakistan	Turkey
Crude birth rate	43	43	34	44	44	44	39
Crude death rate	21	20	13	16	11	15	12
Annual growth rate	2.2	2.3	2.1	2.8	3.2	2.9	2.7
Infant mortality rate	182	169	122	139	99	121	119
Percentage under 15 years of age	44	40	40	47	48	46	42
Life expectancy	40	40	50	51	53	51	57

Source: *1977 World Population Data Sheet,* Population Reference Bureau, Washington, D.C.

is possible. In this section, findings of the three-province survey that increase understanding of rural health problems will be presented.

At the onset of discussion, it should be pointed out that the data on morbidity and mortality were based on the recall of respondents. Numerous studies have demonstrated underreporting of illnesses, especially common childhood ailments, in surveys relying on the recall of informants.[4] Attempts were made to minimize inaccuracies by limiting the period of recall to the immediate 2 weeks before the interview. The survey was carried out from August through October, and therefore illnesses with higher incidences during these months may be overrepresented, while illnesses associated with winter, such as pneumonia, typhus, and common colds, may be underreported. Ideally, morbidity surveys should be repeated in several different seasons, although the increased time and expense involved may outweigh the benefits to the planner.

Another approach to collecting morbidity data is the clinical survey in which the actual signs and symptoms are used as indicators of illness. The need for trained medical staff and the increased expense and higher levels of informant cooperation required decrease the practicality and usefulness of this approach. In addition, the differences in results of the morbidity recall surveys and the clinical surveys previously conducted in rural Afghanistan are not significant, arguing for the lower-cost recall survey employed here.[5]

Illness Prevalence: All female respondents were asked as part of their household interviews if each household member had been sick in the last 2 weeks, the nature of the illness, the treatment sought, and whether the individual was still sick at the time of the interview. Twenty-two percent of household members were reported as having been sick in the 2 weeks prior to the survey; 81.6 percent of those were still sick at interview time. Illnesses reported are summarized in table A–6.

Three types of illnesses, respiratory ailments, gastrointestinal illnesses, and fevers, accounted for 57 percent of all illnesses mentioned. Two illnesses, measles and malnutrition, are notable by their absence. Measles, an illness frequently reported as associated with childhood death, may be low owing to the season, since measles is usually associated with the closer living conditions of the winter months. Malnutrition, which was mentioned in only 0.7 percent of cases, may be underreported because of the fact that it is not perceived as a distinct illness by villagers, but rather an end condition resulting from other health problems. The prevalence of malnutrition as determined by anthropometric measurement is very high, as will be discussed later.

The prevalence of illness, as reported by female respondents, differed by sex, 19.1 percent of males having been reported ill in the last 2 weeks as compared with 24.1 percent of females. While this difference may be attrib-

Table A-6
Illnesses Reported for Household Members in Last 2 Weeks

Illness Reported	Percent of Total (N = 766)	
Respiratory		
Colds	2.7	
Coughs	2.1	
Black cough	0.5	
Pneumonia	3.7	
Tuberculosis	3.2	
Sore throat	0.8	
Other respiratory	5.0	
Subtotal		18.0
Gastrointestinal		
Vomiting	0.8	
Diarrhea	6.9	
Dysentery	4.5	
Cholera	0.4	
Stomach pains	13.6	
Subtotal		26.2
Fevers		
Unspecified	8.8	
Malaria	5.0	
Other	0.8	
Subtotal		14.6
Aches and pains		
Headache	4.5	
Joint pains	3.7	
Arthritis	1.5	
Other pains	11.3	
Subtotal		21.0
Eye problems	1.7	
Women's illnesses	3.8	
All other illnesses	14.7	
Total	100.0	

uted to the fact that informants were women, figure A-4 suggests another hypothesis—namely, that the increased prevalence of illness for females that begins at reproductive ages may in part be a function of the hardships of multiple childbirths.

Figure A-4 also demonstrates that the very young and the old share a disproportionate burden of illness. Possible causes for the high prevalence of illness among the very young will be discussed in the section on nutritional status and childrearing practices.

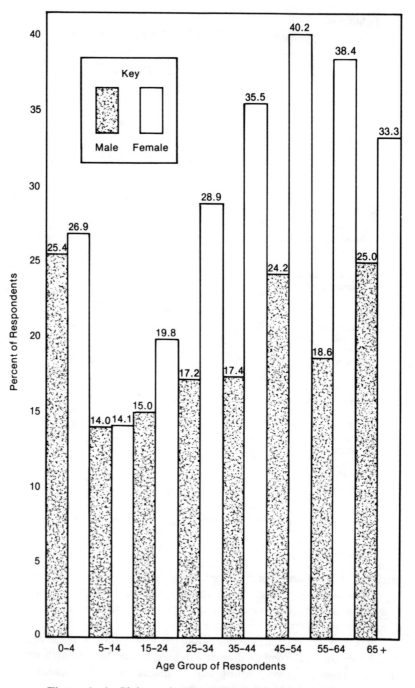

Figure A-4. Sickness in Last 2 Weeks, by Sex and Age

Table A-7
Illnesses Associated with Deaths in the Last Year

Illness	Percent of All Deaths (N = 98)
Pulmonary/respiratory problems	20.4
Dysentery/diarrhea	17.3
Jinns	14.3
Fever	9.2
Swelling	6.1
Measles	3.1
Stomach ache	3.1
Heart disease	3.1
Other	23.4

Table A-8
Illnesses Associated with Deaths of Children Aged 0 to 5 in Last Year

	Age of Death						Percent of Total
	0-1	*1-2*	*2-3*	*3-4*	*4-5*	*Total*	
Jinns	9	0	3	0	0	12	20.7
Diarrhea/ Dysentery	4	5	0	1	1	11	18.9
Pulmonary/ respiratory	2	3	2	0	1	8	13.8
Fever	2	1	2	0	0	5	8.6
Swelling	0	4	1	0	0	5	8.6
Measles	0	1	1	1	0	3	5.2
Other	4	6	1	0	3	14	24.2
Total	21	20	10	2	5	58	
Percent of Total	36.2	34.5	17.2	3.5	8.6	100	100.0

Illnesses Associated with Death: Informants also were asked to describe the illnesses that were associated with each death in the household in the last year. Their responses are listed in table A-7.

The reported causes of death for children from birth to 5 years is presented in table A-8. *Jinns* is a folk classification for childhood deaths attributable to evil spirits with an attraction to the very young. It is difficult to make an exact translation of *jinns* into a specific disease classification, but on the basis of a description of its signs and symptoms and the specific age groups affected, it is tempting to equate *jinns* with neonatal tetanus, especially since neonatal tetanus does not receive any separate mention as a cause of childhood deaths. *Jinns* are often described as convulsions, with a rapid irreversible progression to death, a description compatible with the clinical signs of neonatal tetanus. Surveys done in developing countries report extremely high infant mortality rates owing to tetanus, ranging from 10 percent in Haiti[6] to 54 percent in India.[7] Given the similarity of traditional umbilical-cord severing and care techniques among rural populations, it would be unusual if tetanus were not also an important cause of childhood deaths in Afghanistan. Additionally, 55 percent of the 115 infant deaths reported in the survey and attributed to *jinns* occurred within the first month; this further supports the equation of *jinns* with neonatal tetanus. It is extremely important to verify this association, given the extraordinary reduction in infant death that has been brought about in many countries through low-cost maternal immunization programs.[8] Similarly, the classification of swelling could easily be interpreted as a description of the edema which accompanies malnutrition, and further study should be carried out to determine the interpretation that should be given this classification.

Mothers also were asked to recall the cause of death for all their children who had ever died. Table A–9 summarizes their answers. The large proportion of total child deaths attributed to *jinns* again emphasizes the importance of a further understanding of the exact classification of this illness category. The fact that smallpox appears in table A–9 but not in the listing of causes of death to children in the last year reflects the successful eradication of smallpox in the past 5 years in Afghanistan.

A look at causes of death by age group is instructive. For children aged 0 to 2, *jinns* is the most common cause mentioned. At ages 2 to 3 years, corresponding roughly to the reported age of weaning of Afghan children, diarrhea and dysentery become the leading causes of death.

Most Serious Illnesses as Perceived by Respondents: Both male and female respondents were asked, "In your opinion, what are the most serious illnesses that affect your household and others in your village?" Up to three responses per person were recorded. Table A–9 presents the combined totals for all replies. Interestingly, no respondents reported *jinns* as being the most serious illness, although it was reported as being the single most important cause of child deaths. It may be speculated that while *jinns* kills children, it is not considered as an illness, but rather an action taken by powers beyond the control of medicines and which in the villagers' minds somehow lies beyond the usual classification of illness.

With the exception of *jinns,* there is a strong congruence between those

Table A-9
Illnesses Associated with Total Child Deaths, by Age

Illness	Number of Deaths by Age					Total (N = 701)	Percent of Total
	0-1	1-2	2-3	3-4	4-5		
Jinns	136	35	22	6	8	207	29.6
Pulmonary respiratory	54	25	22	15	4	120	17.0
Diarrhea dysentery	19	17	29	7	6	78	11.2
Measles	11	6	21	12	9	59	8.4
Fever	19	6	10	1	2	38	5.4
Small pox	5	6	10	7	4	32	4.6
Malnutrition	15	0	3	0	0	18	2.6
Injury	6	0	3	1	2	12	1.6
Other	86	14	15	14	8	137	19.6
Total	351	109	135	63	43	701	
Percent of total	50.1	15.5	19.3	9.0	6.1	100	100.0

diseases perceived as most serious and those associated with death. For instance, 32 percent of child deaths in the last year were said to be due to gastrointestinal or respiratory problems, and 56 percent of respondents named these illnesses as being most serious. This has favorable implications for planning village-level health programs, since it is usually easiest to obtain community cooperation and support for a program directed toward a problem that is given priority by the people themselves.

Nutritional Status and Childrearing Practices: Ample evidence of high childhood morbidity and mortality existed in Afghanistan, especially in rural areas, before the design of this survey. One objective of this study was to examine the underlying causes for health problems among the very young, especially related to nutrition and childrearing practices. This section summarizes the information of the nutritional status of children aged 1 to 4 years as determined by measurement of weights, heights, and arm circumferences. Also included is a summary of women's responses to a series of questions designed to obtain information on current childrearing practices in the villages studied.

The first important finding of the study is that there is extensive undernutrition among younger children. Figure A-5 summarizes the results of

Table A-10
Most Serious Illness, All Mentions (Males and Females)

Illness		Percent of Total Mentions
Respiratory illnesses		
Colds	4.8	
Cough	1.1	
Black cough	7.2	
Pneumonia	8.8	
Tuberculosis	8.2	
Sore throat	0.8	
Other	0.2	
Subtotal		31.1
Gastrointestinal illness		
Vomiting	0.7	
Diarrhea	8.6	
Dysentery	11.8	
Cholera	2.4	
Subtotal		23.5
Fevers		
Fever unspecific	8.3	
Malaria	9.0	
Other	3.3	
Subtotal		20.6
Aches and pains		
Stomach ache	3.6	
Headache	2.3	
Other	2.3	
Subtotal		8.2
Measles		7.5
Eye problems		2.0
All others		7.1
		100.0

arm-circumference measurements for 358 children over 1 year and less than 5 years of age. *Well-nourished* has been defined as having an arm circumference in the green, that is, over 13.5 cm measured at middle of the upper arm. All children with red or yellow readings, that is, under 13.5 cm, were exluded from the well-nourished category.

For each age group, the small percentage of children classifiable as well-nourished is striking. For instance, less than 10 percent of children 1 to 3 years old were well-nourished, while of the oldest age group studied (over 4 but less than 5 years of age), less than 60 percent were judged as well-nourished. Table A-11 presents the completed breakdown of arm-circumference statistics by sex and age.

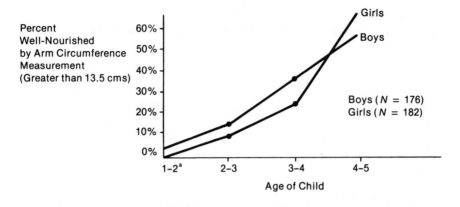

^a In this figure, 1–2 means 1 year old but less than 2 years old, 2–3 means 2 years old but less than 3 years old, and similarly for all other age groups.

Figure A–5. Percentage of Children Classifiable as Well-Nourished

Figure A–5 and table A–11 indicate that girls are less well-nourished than boys up until the age of 4 years, after which they do slightly better than boys. They also demonstrate an overall trend toward less undernutrition in older children than in younger ones. These data must be carefully interpreted, however, for it could be that the decrease is caused by poorly nourished children dying and therefore leaving the sample, as well as from children converting to a well-nourished status with the passage of time.

There can be little doubt about the serious nature of malnutrition in the population studied and undoubtedly in rural Afghanistan in general, even though respondents seldom mention it as a serious health problem. The intersection of malnutrition and other manifestations of illness in Afghanistan can be seen in table A–12, which compares the prevalence of recent illnesses of children classifiable as well-nourished (green) with those definitely malnourished (red).

Malnourished children have a rate of illness almost three times that of children who are well-nourished. This finding does not *prove* that malnutrition causes illness, since it is also possible that it is the illness which causes the child to be malnourished. However, the evidence from this survey as well as numerous other studies[9] is extremely suggestive that poor nutrition leads to increased illness. This has important implications in the design of programs with the objective of child health improvement.

In order to obtain some insight into the nutritional and childrearing behavior of rural women, and perhaps into the cause of nutritional prob-

Table A-11
Arm Circumference (AC), by Age and Sex as Percentage of Total at Each Age

	Green		Yellow		Red	
Age Group	Male	Female	Male	Female	Male	Female
1–2 years	6.1	0.0	33.3	21.2	60.6	78.8
2–3 years	13.7	7.4	58.8	40.7	27.5	51.9
3–4 years	36.2	25.5	51.7	53.2	12.1	21.3
4–5 years	53.4	58.3	33.3	27.1	13.3	14.6

N = 176 males, 182 females

Note: Green: AC > 13.5 cm; Yellow: 12.5 cm ≤ AC ≤ 13.5 cm; Red: AC < 12.5.

Table A-12
Prevalence of Illness in Last 2 Weeks by Nutritional Status of Children over 1 and under 5 Years of Age

		Well-Nourished	Malnourished
Sick in last	Yes	16.7	44.7
2 weeks	No	83.3	55.3

N = 288

lems, each female respondent was asked a set of questions dealing with child-care practices. When asked, "How long do you breast feed your babies?" the mean response of 486 mothers was 2 years, with no significant difference between boys and girls. The relatively long period of breast feeding should be a positive factor in child health; however, it should be remembered that responses were given in terms of ideal breast-feeding lengths. If an event such as pregnancy occurs soon after a birth, it may prove impossible to accomplish the ideal. There was no significant difference in the nutritional status of children measured by arm circumference by the age of weaning reported by their mothers.

Mothers reported giving their children foods in addition to milk at an average age of 11.5 months. Not only is the introduction of solid foods rather late (most experts feel that a child benefits from being given well-prepared solid foods as early as 5 months of age), but the foods currently being introduced are often of marginal value to the growing child. Table A-13 summarizes responses to the question, "What are the best foods to begin feeding your baby?"

Table A-13
Six Best Foods to Introduce to Babies

Food	Percent of Mentions
Rice	19.2
Bread	17.0
Powdered milk	16.6
Bread and tea	6.0
Vegetable soup	4.4
Yogurt	4.2

$N = 452$

Table A-14
Age Reported for Introduction of Specific Foods

Food	Mean Age of Introduction (in Months)
Eggs	26.3
Soft meats	20.2
Vegetables	18.8
Fruits	16.5
Tea	11.5
Bread	11.3

$N = 452$

More instructive than the type of food introduced is the mean age at which respondents reported first giving a particular food to their children, as seen in table A-14. This table contains especially important information. Not only does it indicate one of the underlying causes of poor childhood nutrition—the extremely late reported introduction of high-protein foods into the child's diet—but it also suggests an intervention at the village level with potentially profound implications for child health: improvement of mothers' knowledge of appropriate feeding patterns for small children and modification of current feeding practices. An intervention of this nature could be carried out at low cost, perhaps as part of a Village Health Worker Program, especially if female VHWs were available. Another approach to improving nutritional practice is through the use of mass-media campaigns making use of the radio, an approach that will be discussed in more detail in a later section.

Only 20 percent of the mothers interviewed reported ever giving their children powdered milk, while over 70 percent reported giving animal milk. Frequencies of giving milk were

	Milk Powder	Animal Milk
Never	79.9	28.8
About once per month	0.8	2.3
About once per week	6.5	20.5
Three to four times per week	2.3	7.0
Every day	10.5	41.4

Another factor affecting child nutrition is the prevailing belief about the proper feeding of a sick child. In many societies, food (either all foods or specific foods) is withheld from the sick child. The most common example of this occurs with diarrhea. It is a common belief that solid food, and occasionally liquids as well, should not be given to a child with diarrhea. This frequently leads to undernutrition, weakness, and dehydration. Both men and women in the sample were asked, "Should you feed your child when he has diarrhea?" One-third of the men and one-quarter of the women stated that a child with diarrhea should not be given food. In addition, men were asked whether water should be given. Over 20 percent reported that it should not be. Among those stating that a child with diarrhea should be fed, soft rice was the food most frequently suggested.

There is much about the nutrition of children in the Afghan village that this survey was unable to learn. Questions such as How much food is available to the household? What foods are actually given to small children? How are they fed? How often? How is food distributed among the household members? are important questions, and ones that could be answered only by more detailed nutritional surveys. They are questions that must be answered, however, if village-level health programs are going to be designed to meet the most basic health problems facing rural people.

Attitudes Toward Family Size: Essential to learning about the feasibility of using child spacing as an element of a general rural health program is an understanding of the attitudes of couples toward the number of children they want, as well as their interest in learning about ways to increase the time between births.

Increased birth intervals allow a mother to give a child more of her time and attention, since she will not have several small children to care for simultaneously. The child will receive extended breast feeding. A greater

space between children usually means fewer births during a woman's reproductive period, and thus family resources are divided among fewer persons.
Most important, a women's health will be improved with longer rest
between children, and her ability to care for the children she does have will
be improved.

Both men and women were asked how many additional children they
would like to have. Sixty-three percent of the men and 65 percent of the
women said that they would like to have no more children. The mean number of additional children desired was 1.27, with boys being more desired
than girls by a ratio of approximately 2:1. The number of additional children desired by women is shown in table A–15.

Not unexpectedly, the number of additional children desired decreases
with the number of living children a woman already has. A single exception
to this trend occurs among women with no living children who desire fewer
"additional" children than women with one to two living children. This
inconsistency is explained by the fact that one-half of the twenty women in
the sample with no children were over 35 years old. These women most
likely were incapable of producing any children and therefore would not
express an anticipation of having any additional children. There was no
association between the number of children who had died and the number
of additional children that a woman desired. The number of additional children also shows a direct inverse relationship to the age of female respondents, as shown in table A–16.

Table A–15
Additional Children Desired, by Number of Living Children of Female Respondents

Number of Living Children	Mean Number of Additional Children Desired
0	2.45
1	3.20
2	2.92
3	1.53
4	0.74
5	0.64
6	0.46
7	0.17

$N = 333$

Table A-16
Mean Number of Additional Children Wanted, by Age of Female
Respondent

Age of Female	Mean Number of Additional Children Wanted
15–19	3.91
20–24	2.96
25–29	2.47
30–34	1.53
35–39	0.98
40–44	0.64
45–49	0.50
N = 333	

As noted earlier in the discussion of fertility, the number of children born to women in rural Afghanistan now and in the past is extremely high; women aged 15 to 19 years will have 9.2 children by the time they have completed their reproduction if current rates of fertility continue. The average desired family size, the number of living children plus additional children desired, is also high, as might be expected.

Nonetheless, 69 percent of the males and 91.6 percent of the females interviewed stated that they would be "interested in learning about ways that would allow them to increase the amount of time between pregnancies." The number of women expressing an interest in learning about spacing methods is especially noteworthy and carries implications for the services that could be productively provided by a village health worker.

The Village Environment: The environmental condition of a village is another factor in illness. Poor sanitation, crowding, lack of proper water supply, and inadequate housing all contribute to morbidity and mortality in the Afghan village.

As discussed earlier, the average rural household consists of slightly over seven persons living in 2.25 rooms, or just over three persons per room. Such conditions lead to the rapid spread of infectious diseases, especially during winter seasons when families spend more time gathered together in the home. Sharing facilities with livestock also increases the risk of animal-borne vector diseases.

All male respondents also were asked the source of the drinking water used by their household. Sources mentioned were

Jui (open irrigation ditch)	37% (*N* = 198)
Well in yard	23%
Karez (underground tunnels)	19%
Spring	13%
River	6%
Well in village	2%

Seventy-eight percent of men reported being satisfied with their source of drinking water. Nonetheless, 86 percent said that they would be willing to contribute their labor to improve the drinking supply to their village if government specialists were available for technical assistance; 60 percent reported a willingness to contribute money to the same cause.

The primary sanitation facility used by the households sampled were

Latrine in yard	41.8%
No facility	27.7%
Deep hole outside yard	15.8%
Deep hole in yard	4.5%
Latrine in house	4.0%
Other facilities	6.2%

Fewer men, only 55 percent, were satisfied with their sanitation facilities. Eighty-one percent of male respondents claimed a readiness to contribute labor to improve their sanitation, and almost 50 percent would contribute money for the purpose of improving village sanitation facilities.

There is an apparent need for improvement of the environmental conditions in rural villages. Some of these improvements, such as the wholesale improvement in housing, will prove extremely difficult. Others may be accomplished more easily, especially given the strong inclination of informants to help themselves if technical assistance were available from governmental sources.

Socioeconomic Status of Households and Health Problems: The economic status of a household often affects the health of its members. For instance, in this survey, 41.9 percent of children aged 1 to 4 years in households characterized as very poor were classified as being malnourished, compared with 21.0 percent in households that were average or better. In the households classified as average or better, 38.7 percent of the children were classified as well-nourished, compared with only 27.7 percent in very poor households.

Women in very poor households have both greater numbers of children who had died and a larger number of children living than do women in households with an SES of average or better:

SES	Living Children	Children Died	Desired Total Family Size
Very poor	4.3	1.92	6.9
Average or better	3.7	1.85	5.9

Significantly, women in the lowest SES classification had a desired total family size, that is, living children plus additional children wanted, that was one child larger than those in the highest SES category. While it is not possible in this book to analyze all data by SES, these findings support the conclusion demonstrated by innumerable studies and surveys around the world: poverty is accompanied by increased risks of poor health, higher mortality, and an accompanying trend toward increased fertility rates. The implication of this is that any health program, to be effective, must be designed in such a way as to reach those in the greatest need, most frequently including the very poorest segment of the population.

Rural Health Resources

Every society evolves methods to promote and maintain the health of its members. To those concerned with the planning and management of health programs, an appreciation of the existing health resources is as important as an understanding of the nature of the health problems facing a community. In this section, the health-seeking behavior of rural villages will be described. As described in an earlier MOPH report,[10] the alternatives that a villager has available in the event of an illness, or to ward off sickness, are many. While the entire system of health services, both modern and traditional, is too complex to describe here, (see appendix B), there are general statements that can be made:

The present network of health resources in rural Afghanistan is composed of many layers of belief, tradition, and practice.

The villager is, above all, pragmatic in the way that he or she seeks care. Several different sources of expertise may be drawn upon for a single episode of illness, with little energy being expended in attributing cures to one specific source or another.

The new and the old in health care exist comfortably side by side in rural Afghanistan. Traditions of curing tend to be more accumulative than competitive. For the same reasons that an individual will seek advice from several different sources when sick, the advent of modern treatments has not eliminated the existence of more traditional practices and practitioners.

The household represents the first, and in many cases the primary, source of care for most rural Afghans when sick. Treatment is usually sought beyond the household only after knowledge and treatments available in the family home have proven inadequate for the problem.

The decision as to the type of treatment to be sought after home treatment proves inadequate is a complex one involving numerous considerations such as the perceived cause and severity of the illness, the age and sex of the individual, the amount of money available to the family, the availability of transport, and the household's past experience with similar illnesses.

The findings of the three-province survey provide extensive information on the behavior of rural households in pursuing health, as well as the amount of money expended. Figure A–6 is a map of health resources that attempts to convey both the complexity of the network of services available and their spatial relationship to the household, and it serves here as the focal point for the analysis of health needs and health behavior. Appendix B includes a brief description of each of the sources of health care appearing in figure A–6.

Sources of Treatment: An analysis of the type of treatment sought for the 740 household members who were reported as having been sick in the last 2 weeks provides one measure of the health-seeking behavior of the populations studied. Of those reported to have been sick, 496, or 67 percent, reported having used at least one specific treatment. The average number of treatments mentioned for those who did seek care was 1.55, with 15 percent having tried three or more different sources of treatment. The sources of treatment and the frequency with which they were used are presented in table A–17.

Table A–17 affirms that the single most frequent source of treatment for illness is the household itself, primarily herbal remedies, food prescription and proscription, prayer, and bed rest. Also important is that the Basic Health Center was reported to have been used in 25 percent of all illnesses and was the single most frequently consulted source of treatment outside the home. This is an indication of the important role now being played by the BHC; this also suggests the potential of the BHC to perform an even

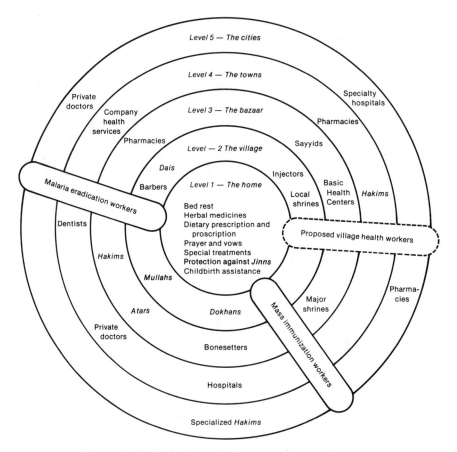

Figure A-6. Overview of Afgan Rural Health Resources

larger role in the delivery of services. Other than for the *mullah,* reported use of traditional services was low, but underreporting is a possibility, since interviewers were clearly perceived by villagers as being advocates of modern types of treatment—a bias impossible to avoid when highly literate interviewers are required.

The sources of treatment sought for all deaths in the last year provide information on the types of care sought in life-threatening situations rather than for the more common illnesses. Thirty-eight percent of those who died had received no treatment; 27 percent had consulted three or more different sources. An average of 1.9 sources were consulted per death. The sources consulted are summarized in table A-18.

Not surprisingly, the sources of treatment sought for household members who died show an increased usage of sources of care more special-

Table A-17
Frequency of Use of Sources of Treatment for Illness in Last 2 Weeks

Treatment Used	Percent of Illness for which Used
Home treatment	58.8
Basic Health Center	25.4
Private doctor (local)	12.9
Hospital (regional)	12.5
Private Doctor (regional)	9.6
Pharmacy	9.0
Bazaar	8.2
Private doctor (Kabul)	5.2
Mullah	4.8
Dokhan	3.8
Hospital (Kabul)	2.4
Treatment outside country	1.2
Malaria specialist	0.6
Hakimji	0.4
Cupper	0.2

Table A-18
Frequency of Use of Sources of Treatment for Deaths in Last Year

Treatment Used	Percent of Deaths for which Used (N = 61)
Private doctor (regional)	37.7
Home treatment	32.8
Basic Health Center	26.2
Mullah	24.5
Hospital (regional)	19.6
Private doctor (local)	14.7
Pharmacy	14.7
Private doctor (Kabul)	9.8
Hospital (Kabul)	3.2
Dokhan	3.2

ized, more expensive, and at greater distance from the village. Treatment at the health center was sought for 25 percent of all persons who died, again showing the important role the health center plays, especially for villagers living within 10 or 15 km of a Basic Health Center.

In the year prior to the survey, households sampled made an average of 17.5 visits to all sources of medical care, with a mean of 3.63 different sources consulted per household. Table A-19 summarizes the percentage of households reporting to have used specific sources of treatment as well as the median number of visits for households that used the sources.

This table clearly demonstrates the wide variety of resources utilized by rural populations and supports the view that villages do not use one system of care, modern or traditional, to the exclusion of another. Almost 60 percent of respondents had used a pharmacy in the previous year; 50 percent had visited a Basic Health Center, but almost 50 percent also visited a *mullah* and 25 percent made a visit to a shrine for an illness. Several traditional sources, however, appear to be relied on only infrequently, particularly the cupper and the barber.

Both men and women were asked specifically whether anyone in their households had ever used a Basic Health Center. Fifty-one percent of the men and 67 percent of the women reported having done so. There appear to be only slight differences in the use of the BHC by distance:

Distances from BHC to Village	Percent of Women Having Used BHC
1 km	75 ($N = 476$)
10 km	61
15 km	63

Those who had not used the BHC gave the reasons shown in table A-20.

Very few respondents mentioned the distance to the BHC as a reason for not using its services, while the fact that money is required for services was mentioned often as a reason why men did not use the services. Approximately 25 percent of households reported using the village shop, or *dokhan,* as a source of medicine in the prior year. Their overall opinion of the quality of medicine they were able to obtain from the *dokhan* was not high, however. Only 26.8 percent of respondents considered the medicines to be "good."

Male respondents were asked whether they get advice from anyone outside their household when a family member was sick. Only 15 percent of respondents answered that they did. The person who gave the advice was almost always reported as being another man living in the same village. Only infrequently, less than 25 percent of cases, were these sources said to dispense medicines as well as advice. However, 58 percent of women and 37 percent of men knew of someone in their own village who could give them an injection if needed. In less than 15 percent of the cases was the injectionist described as a person who also dispensed medicines.

Pregnancy and childbirth are recognized in all societies as times of potential physical and emotional problems. Not surprisingly, a specialist

Table A-19
Percentage of Population Using Various Sources of Treatment, per
Median Number of Visits

Source	Households Using	Median Number of Visits
Pharmacy	59.1	3.19
BHC	49.8	1.98
Mullah	48.5	3.28
Injectionist	28.7	5.40
Shrine	26.6	1.40
Doctor (regional)	26.2	2.35
Dokhan	23.6	7.50
Hospital (regional)	20.7	2.13
Atar	12.7	3.50
Doctor (Kabul)	12.7	1.33
Dai (midwife)	11.8	1.20
Doctor (local)	11.0	3.50
Hakimji	10.1	2.25
Barber	6.8	1.39
Bonesetter	5.9	1.14
Hospital (Kabul)	5.5	1.15
Cupper	1.7	1.50
(N = 237)		

Table A-20
Reasons for Not Using BHC, Male and Female Respondents

Reason	Male (N = 98)	Female (N = 143)
No one sick	46.9	27.5
Services in town better	7.1	10.5
No medicines available at BHC	6.1	7.7
Staff require money	16.3	7.7
Family objection	0.0	7.0
Too far away	1.0	7.3
Go to private doctor	0.0	5.6
Heard bad things about BHC	4.1	0.0

source of care is common for this particular problem. Slightly less than 50 percent of female respondents reported using a traditional midwife, or *dai*, for their deliveries. Most *dais* used (89 percent) were located in the same village as the respondent. Of those not using a *dai*, the vast majority (93 percent) relied on female relatives for delivery assistance. All women, regardless of the type of help they reported receiving for childbirth, were asked whether they were satisfied with the services available. Their responses were

Response	Percent	
Very satisfied	6.6	
Satisfied	50.8	$(N = 470)$
Intermediate	30.9	
Unsatisfied	8.9	
Very unsatisfied	2.8	

The fact that only 11 percent of women rated their childbirth assistance as unsatisfactory is evidence that the methods evolved for handling normal deliveries in the village meet the needs of most women as they perceive them.

Cost of Health Services: As important as the information on the types of services being utilized is the amount of money that rural householders pay for the services they receive. Household health-expenditure data are useful in obtaining a better understanding of the marketplace for health care and to determine the financial capacity of villages to support new programs designed to improve their health.

It has been estimated that the per capita annual government health expenditure is approximately 20 Afghanis.[11] It is obvious that even if the MOPH budget were spread equitably over the entire population of the country, there would be severe limitations on the services that could be provided to the country's 23,000 villages if only Ministry resources were utilized. However, the median annual personal health expenditure, according to male informants, is 139 Afghanis or almost seven times the government expenditure.

Data on household incomes in rural Afghanistan is scarce and of questionable accuracy. However, if the mean annual household income of 13,600 Afghanis (which was obtained from a 1971 survey of 254 farmers in Parwan and Ghazni[12]) is considered representative of rural Afghanistan in general, health expenditures are 7.4 percent of the annual household income.

Table A–21 summarizes how male informants reported allocating their household health budget of approximately 1,000 Afghanis per year. These data present a wealth of information on the health behavior of rural Afghans. For example, they vividly point out that the single highest expenditures is for the purchase of medicines at the pharmacy, 37 percent of the

Table A-21
Health Expenditures, by Source and Average Cost of Services

Source	Percent of Health Expenditure	Average Paid Per Visit (in Afghanis)[a]
Pharmacy	37.0	248
Hospital (regional)	12.1	327
Doctor (regional)	9.0	182
Doctor (Kabul)	8.0	664
Basic Health Center	5.7	54
Dokhan	4.6	36
Hospital (Kabul)	4.4	909
Mullah	4.0	33
Shrine	3.5	122
Other (includes care outside the country)	2.8	958
Injectionist	2.4	14
Hakimji	2.4	85
Doctor (local)	1.7	45
Atar	1.0	32
Dai	0.9	94
Bonesetter	0.2	47
Barber	0.2	30
Cupper	0.1	39

[a] Includes transportation costs (50 Afghanis = $1.00)

total health budget. They also demonstrate the extremely high cost of a pharmacy visit (average cost 248 Afghanis) relative to most other sources of treatment.

These data also demonstrate that an illness requiring care in Kabul, either from a private physician or a hospital, is a major expense. This was underlined by a statement of one respondent when asked what people in his village do for an illness too serious to be treated at home: "Those who are lucky enough to have money go to Kabul for help. Those like many of us who have no money must stay in the village and either get better or die." Table A-21 also confirms the wide variety of treatment sources employed. Note that even though visit payments for a traditional practitioner are considerably less than for a modern service, villagers spend almost 20 percent of their health budget on traditional treatments. Additionally, the data demonstrate that a visit to a Basic Health Center often requires some expense, either for transportation or services.

In summary, the health-expenditure data imply that since villagers are already spending large amounts of money for health services, in absolute as well as relative terms, any plan that calls for villagers themselves to contribute to the support of a local health program could be successful as long as villagers perceive the program as being beneficial and worthy of their support. This could have immediate implications for the planning of the new Village Health Worker Program. One additional factor should be kept in mind, however. While the median household health expenditure is very high, over 25 percent of the households spent less than 100 Afghanis for health care. In order to plan programs that will reach all those in need, it would be essential to understand whether these households had no one in the household who was sick during the year or whether they represent a segment of the population that simply did not have the money to spend.

Attitudes toward Available Health Resources: Another important factor in planning health programs is the attitude of villagers toward the services presently available. Logically, there will be greater interest in and cooperation with a program designed to improve services considered unsatisfactory than for one that deals with services that are currently satisfactorily meeting the needs of the village. All female respondents were asked whether they were satisfied with the source of treatment for household members who had been sick in the last 2 weeks. Table A-22 summarizes their responses.

All respondents also were asked where they felt they received the best treatment for an illness that could not be treated at home. Table A-23 summarizes their replies. Both men and women mentioned the Basic Health Center most frequently as the best source of treatment. Other than for the

Table A-22
Satisfaction, by Source of Treatment, Female Respondents

Source	Percent Satisfied (N = 468)
Private doctor (local)	75.0
Hospital (regional)	71.0
Basic Health Center	64.7
Bazaar	57.9
Private doctor (Kabul)	57.1
Private doctor (regional)	53.5
Pharmacy	52.4
Mullah	52.4
Home	49.6
Dokhan	31.6

BHC, there was little agreement between men and women on the best source of treatment. Men tended to name sources in the cities as best, while women selected sources near to home. For instance, 29 percent of men, but only 3 percent of women thought hospitals in Kabul were best, while 25 percent of the women and only 5.3 percent of the men named the *mullah* or shrine. This undoubtedly reflects the greater mobility of men, travel to the cities being a more realistic possibility for them than for women.

Those who reported having used the Basic Health Center were asked their opinion on the quality of the medicine and services they received. Responses indicated a broad range of attitudes:

Quality of Medicines and Services at BHC	Percentage of Males (140)	Percentage of Females (291)
Very good	7.9	11.0
Good	50.0	48.5
Intermediate	17.8	16.5
Poor	23.6	23.7
Very poor	0.7	0.3

The general feeling about the services provided by the BHC is a favorable one, even though almost one-fourth of respondents gave poor ratings. A similar distribution of responses was given when the question was asked concerning the personal treatment received from BHC staff, with slightly fewer poor replies.

Table A-23
Most Frequently Named Best Source of Treatment Outside Home

	Percent Response	
Best Treatment	Males (N = 227)	Females (N = 468)
Basic Health Center	34.8	33.3
Hospital (Kabul)	29.1	3.0
Private doctor (regional)	8.8	14.5
Private doctor (Kabul)	7.0	2.6
Regional hospital	7.0	6.4
Mullah or shrine	5.3	25.0
Private doctor (local)	3.1	8.8
Village	2.6	0
Pharmacy	.9	3.4

Personal Treatment Received at BHC	Percentage of Males (141)	Percentage of Females (283)
Very good	11.3	11.7
Good	58.9	53.3
Intermediate	14.9	17.7
Poor	9.9	7.7
Very poor	5.0	0.0

Several questions were asked to determine whether respondents perceived any improvement in health conditions in the past few years. The first was "Do you feel that children are healthier or less healthy than 5 years ago?" The responses were as follows:

	Males (223)	Females (430)
Healthier	63.7	38.6
Same	15.7	23.5
Less healthy	20.6	37.9

Apparently women are less favorably impressed with present health conditions than men, the same percentage saying that children are less healthy than in the past. The reasons the respondents gave for their responses are listed in table A–24.

Similarly women were somewhat less positive than men about improvements in child mortality in the last 5 years. When asked "Do you think that more or fewer children die now than 5 years ago?" they responded:

	Male Respondents (204)	Female Respondents (421)
More die now	11.7	28.3
Same	21.6	14.5
Fewer die now	66.7	57.2

The final question was whether respondents felt that health services had improved in the last 5 years. Almost 75 percent of all respondents felt that health services were better now than they were 5 years ago. The overall attitude of respondents appears to be that general health conditions have improved in recent years. The implications of this for change in the attitudes of parents toward the number of children they desire is important. It has been hypothesized that parents will seek to control the number of children they have only if they have assurance that the children that they do

Table A-24
Reasons Given for Current Child Health Status, Male Respondents

Reasons Given for Poorer Child Health	*Percent (N = 33)*
More children now	39.3
More disease	30.3
Bad weather	9.0
Bad health services	9.0
Poverty	3.0
Bad water	3.0
Medicines not free	3.0
More malaria	3.0
Other	0.4
Reasons Given for Improved Child Health	*Percent (N = 112)*
Medicine and doctor available	52.6
Less disease	12.5
God's help	8.5
Good weather	8.5
Better food	5.1
Hospital	4.1
Cleanliness improved	4.1
Transportation	2.8
Other	1.8

have have an increased probability of survival.[13] The survey, however, did not demonstrate any significant differences in fertility or desired family size by respondents' perceptions of improvements in health services or child "survivability."

However, among women who had three or more children who have died, there is somewhat less interest in contraception than among women who have not lost any children:

	Number of Children Died	
	0 (N = 123)	*3 or more (N = 71)*
Interested in contraception	16%	5%
Not interested in contraception	84%	95%

It is premature to predict whether perceptions of villagers about child survivability are changing substantially enough to have a significant impact on the number of children desired. In a situation such as in Afghanistan, where 38 percent of women sampled have had more than three children die and several respondents had as many as ten children die, there may be a considerable time lag before actual fertility patterns change in accordance with feelings of the chances of a child surviving to adulthood. It is a subject that requires continued study.

All respondents were asked what in their opinion was the most needed health improvement in their village. Table A-25 compiles their most frequent responses.

This information is useful because it shows that villagers are more concerned with having improved access to medicines than they are in better health facilities or physicians. This was also seen in table A-22, which showed fewer people satisfied with pharmacies and *dokhans* than with most other health services available.

Access to medicines may be limited by cost as much as by the distances to pharmacies or the supply of medicines stocked. As shown earlier, medicines are the single most expensive item in the health budget of rural Afghans, both on an annual and a per visit basis. The priority given to having access to medicines may be a very favorable factor in the success of any village-level program whose objective is to increase the availability of essential, low-cost medicines, whether it is through village health centers, village shops, or pharmacies.

Attitudes of Villagers toward the Feasibility of a VHW Program: One approach to the expansion of health services in rural areas is the village health worker, a concept that has been successfully introduced in a number of countries. One of the objectives of this survey was to determine the receptivity of rural Afghans to the idea of an individual from their village being recruited, trained, and supervised to manage the most common health problems of the village.

In order to learn villagers' views on the feasibility of a Village Health Worker Program, all respondents were asked "In some countries persons from villages have been trained to treat the most common health problems facing the people of their village. Do you feel that this type of thing could be possible for your village?" As can be seen below, reaction was strongly positive for the feasibility of such a program:

	Males (235)	*Females (483)*
Feasible	78.3%	95.3%
Not feasible	17.4%	3.7%
Don't know	4.3%	1.0%

Of those stating that such a program would not be feasible for their village, the most common reason given (60 percent of all replies) was that there was no one in their village qualified for the role. Questions designed to

Table A-25
Most-Needed Health Improvements

Most-Needed Improvement	Percent of Mentions (N = 1241)
Medicines	30.5
Doctor	24.4
Hospital	10.5
Improved sanitation	8.9
Better food	7.5
Transportation and roads	2.6

elicit information about which characteristics would be most important for a person who would serve as a village health worker produced the responses shown in table A-26.

This table points out that both men and women felt that it would be important that women be trained as VHWs. It also shows that personal qualities such as good character and proper attitude are judged to be more important qualifications than experience or intellect, even though respondents share the common belief that candidates should be literate. While literacy is rated highly and respondents felt that VHWs should have at least 10 years of education, whether or not such qualifications are either essential or useful for such a role is unclear, especially since some studies have shown that the most successful change agents at the village level are persons who share as many characteristics as possible with the people they serve.[14] Persons of higher education may automatically be distinguished from the majority of villagers and may be less successful as change agents then persons less well educated. The important question is what is the minimal education required in order to perform the specific tasks.

Respondents also were asked how they felt VHWs should be selected. Replies were as follows:

	Males (N = 182)	Females (N = 438)
By the people	47.3%	42.3%
By the government	39.7%	40.2%
By village leaders	7.7%	11.9%
By the government and people	3.5%	2.3%
By leaders and people	0.6%	1.6%
From among the injectionists in the village	0.6%	1.7%

Table A-26
Best Characteristics for Village Health Workers

	Percent Replies	
	Male (N = 193)	Female (N = 421)
Best Age for a VHW [a]		
Young	30.0	42.3
Middle-aged	26.3	24.9
Older	6.3	4.6
Don't know	37.4	28.2
Best Sex for VHWs		
Male	13.7	11.6
Female	6.3	43.3
Both	80.0	45.1
Should Literacy be Required?		
Yes	100.0	81.3
Should VHW Have Experience Outside Village?		
Yes	94.3	98.4
What Are Best Qualifications for VHWs? (Most Frequent Responses Only)		
Good character and patience	40.4	54.4
Proper manner	15.3	2.6
Humanitarian	10.4	4.5
Experience	8.2	1.0
Intelligence	6.6	26.0

[a] N = 190 for men, 494 for women

The most common belief was that the people of the village should themselves decide who should be their village health worker. However, large segments of the population also stated the opposing viewpoint, that the government should make the selection, indicating that the best method might vary from village to village and might realistically depend on the specific political structure encountered as much as on the attitudes of the people. Interestingly, the question brought forth a suggestion from a small number of respondents that is worthy of consideration, namely, that those in the village currently in roles where they provide a health service for the village, such as injectionists, should be given first consideration for the VHW role. This may prove to be a suggestion worth pursuing.

Twenty-six percent of males and 18 percent of females could think of a specific person in their village who they felt would make a good VHW. In

Table A-27
Characteristics of Persons Nominated for VHW Role

	Males (N = 59)	Females (N = 79)
Mean age	33.5 years	31.5 years
Sex: Male	91.4 percent	61.8 percent
Female	8.6 percent	38.2 percent
Education: Mean years	9.2 years	7.9 years
Literacy	82.8 percent	72.0 percent
Experience outside village	63.8 percent	61.5 percent

Table A-28
Reasons Given for Nomination of Individual as VHW

	Percent of Males (N = 62)	Percent of Females (N = 98)
People like him/her	35	27
Good education	19	14
Person is informed	15	7
Person is clever	13	35
Person is useful	13	5
Knows how to give injections	5	1
Relative of respondent	0	11

those cases in which an individual was nominated, their characteristics had the profile shown in table A-27.

One of the problems anticipated in establishing a VHW Program has been the lack of qualified women. Table A-27 is encouraging in that over 33 percent of females responding were able to nominate a woman from the village who they thought would make a good VHW. Also encouraging is that 27 percent of male respondents stated that they would allow their wives or daughters to be trained as village health workers.

Thirty percent of males but only 10 percent of females felt that it would be possible to find a woman from the village to be trained as a VHW if training were nearby and she could return home in the evenings. Somewhat surprisingly, slightly more (34 percent of males) answered affirmatively when the same question was asked, but training was described as being farther away, requiring women to spend an extended period away from the village. There was a slight drop in positive replies among women for these conditions. Respondents also were asked why they nominated the person they did for the VHW role. Their replies are shown in table A-28. Again, the belief that a good character is a more desired characteristic than knowledge or experience in selecting a VHW appears to be supported, especially in responses of males.

Over 200 male respondents were asked whether VHWs would have to be paid. Eighty percent felt that they would. The following methods of payment were suggested:

People should provide salary	43%	
Government should provide salary	27%	
People could not provide salary	20%	47% other than villagers themselves
People provide part of salary	10%	

Men were obviously divided on whether or not the village would be able to support a VHW. The answer to the question of whether a village can or will support a VHW will come from actual experience and may well differ from area to area. The percentage of men that thought the village itself could pay for the health worker varied from 100 to 22 percent in villages studied. The method by which payment is collected also may make a difference. For instance, villagers may be reluctant to join an insurance scheme to help pay for the support of a VHW whether or not there is anyone in their house-hold requiring his or her service, but they may be readily willing to buy medicines from a VHW knowing that he or she will receive a small profit from each sale.

The method by which a VHW will be supported is a key question, especially since one major assumption of the Ministry of Public Health's planned program is that the village health worker would be nearly self-sufficient and operate with minimal government expenditures beyond those incurred for training and supervision.

Diffusion of Information in Rural Villages: As described earlier, many of the health problems in the rural populations studied, especially those of small children, arise from lack of information as much as from lack of available health services. The nutrition of children, treatment of the umbilicus of newborns leading to tetanus, and the treatment used for diarrhea are important examples of health problems caused or exacerbated by lack of knowledge.

One remedy is obvious—increased information. However, before beginning a program aimed at improving health education, it is essential to have an understanding of channels by which villagers, especially women who are the prime targets, currently receive information. The question posed is an immense one, and one that the three-province survey has only begun to investigate.

All women interviewed were asked whether they ever listen to the radio.

Table A–29
Frequency of Radio Listening by Women Who Listen

Times per Week Listened	Percent of Responses (N = 245)
< 1	13.5
1	4.1
2	11.0
3	5.7
4	1.2
5	0.4
6	1.6
7 or more	62.4

Almost 50 percent reported that they did, and table A–29 records their reported frequency of listening.

Two-thirds of women listeners reported having radios in their homes; most of the rest listened in the homes of friends or relatives. The most interesting programs, as reported by women listeners, were

Music	62.1%
Family life	19.4%
News	9.7%
Farmer's program	3.7%
Stories	2.8%
Radio doctor	2.3%

Men were asked a slightly different question, namely: "How many days a week do you listen to the radio?" Their responses are shown in table A–30. Their favorite programs were reported to be

News	32.7%
Farmer's program	27.1%
Music	19.6%
Radio doctor	7.5%
Family life	5.6%
Stories	1.9%

The radio is one of the major means by which new ideas come into the village. Information on the radio listening habits of men and women has

Table A-30
Frequency of Radio Listening by All Men

Days. per-Week Listened	Percent of Responses
0	61.2
1	5.1
2	2.1
3	2.5
4	.8
5	2.5
6	1.3
7	24.5

broad implications for health-education programs. The first fact is that the percentage of people in the village who have access to a radio is extremely high. Second, women report listening to the radio as frequently as men, if not more frequently. There are, however, distinct differences in the favorite programs of men and women. Women rate music programs as their overwhelming favorite, while men report favoring the news and farmers' program. Neither men nor women rate the radio doctor program among their favorites.

There are several important implications in these findings. First, the radio would have the possibility of reaching a very large percentage of the rural population with health-education messages. Second, these health messages would be most effective if sent via the most listened-to program, that is, music for health education messages for women and news or farmers' programs for messages for men. One of the most successful campaigns to improve the nutrition of rural children has been carried out in Zambia, a country with geographic and language barriers similar to Afghanistan's. The approach used has relied heavily on popular radio programs and nutrition messages incorporated into popular music. In fact, in most years, the most popular song has been a message on nutrition or childrearing produced by the National Nutrition Commission. The potential for this type of health-education program in rural Afghanistan is extremely favorable, given the radio-listening habits of the rural population.

Another potential use of the radio that should be mentioned is in communicating with VHWs dispersed around the country to provide them with ongoing information, instructions, and encouragement. One example of this approach is the Nigerian extension workers' "Radio Farmer." This is a program broadcast on national radio once a week, to which all extension workers listen to find out what other workers are doing and to upgrade their own knowledge. Such an approach also might work well for village health workers.

Another means by which information diffuses into the village is by villagers who travel to regional centers and to the cities. As was already shown for the source of treatment used by men and women, there is a great difference in mobility according to sex. All the men were asked whether they permit their wives to go to the following places alone:

Place	Percentage Permitting (N = 230)
Visiting female friends in village	41.8
Bazaar	7.8
Basic Health Center	12.9
Shrine in village	6.5

When women were asked whether they were allowed to travel outside the household alone they gave the following replies:

Place	Percentage Allowed (N = 431)
Visiting female friends in village	3.3
Bazaar	6.7
Basic Health Center	44.3
Shrine in village	19.0

This information points out the severe limitations on women's movement outside the household. The small percentage of women reporting being allowed to visit female friends in the village points out the restrictions on the spread of information from woman to woman within the village.

The Basic Health Center, however, appears to represent a force for change. The ability of greater percentages of women to travel to the health center than to other places makes it an advantageous site for the spread of information both from health center staff to those attending and from woman to woman. Programs should be arranged at the BHC to take advantage of this opportunity.

The current channels of communication to the rural Afghan woman are quite narrow; the potential for their expansion, making use of innovative health-education programs, is, however, great.

Socioeconomic Status and Health Behavior: Just as the SES of a household can affect the health of its members, so too can socioeconomic status be an important determinant of both what a household does when one of its members is sick and the access that a family has to information. As discussed earlier, while the average amount a rural household pays for health care annually is quite high, there are many households in which expenditures are very low. Analysis shows that the health expenditure of very poor households is approximately one-half that of households above average. Furthermore, attitudes as to the best treatment for illness appear to vary by socioeconomic category as well. For instance, 34 percent of poor women felt that the *mullah* offered the best care when sick, while only 15 percent of the average or above-average households mentioned this source. Likewise, 16 percent of average or above average women felt that a hospital was the best place to go when sick, compared with 3 percent of very poor women. Slightly fewer (24 percent) of average or above average women perceived the BHC as providing the best care, as did very poor women (40 percent). There was no difference by SES for receptivity to the concept of a village health worker. Not surprisingly, poor women have considerably less access to a radio and therefore could be expected to be reached less easily by that means than women in households that are wealthier and possess their own radios.

While not all differences between the rich and the poor are significant or important for the planning of health services, the specific needs and constraints of the poor must be taken into consideration in planning village health schemes.

Notes

1. Alfred A. Buck; Robert I. Anderson; K. Kawata; I.W. Abrahams; R.A. Ward; and T.T. Sasaki, *Health and Disease in Rural Afghanistan* (Baltimore, Md.: York Press, 1972); WHO, *Infant and Early Childhood Mortality Survey* (Institute of Public Health, Kabul, 1974); CINAM, *Services for Children within Regional Development Lines* (UNICEF, Kabul, 1973); and Management Sciences for Health, *A Field Survey of Health Needs Practices and Resources in Rural Afghanistan* (Cambridge, Mass.: MSH, 1975).

2. Management Sciences for Health, *A Proposed Village Health Worker Program for Afghanistan* (Cambridge, Mass.: MSH, 1977).

3. Central Statistics Office, *National Demographic and Family Guidance Survey of the Settled Population of Afghanistan* (Kabul, Afghanistan: CSO, 1975).

4. Reynaldo Martorell; Jean-Pierre Habicht; C. Arbrough; A Lechtig; and R.E. Klein, "Underreporting in Fortnightly Recall Morbidity Surveys," *Environmental Child Health* (1976):129–132.

5. Buck, *Health and Disease;* and WHO, *Infant and Early Childhood Mortality Survey.*

6. A.M. Earle and W.L. Mellon, *American Journal of Tropical Medicine and Hygiene* (1958):315–317.

7. S.M.H. Jaffari, et al., *Indian Pediatrics,* 3(1966):177–182.

8. John K. Miller, "The Prevention of Neonatal Tetanus by Maternal Immunization," *Environmental Child Health* (1972):160–170.

9. Carl E. Taylor, N.S. Scrimshaw, and John E. Gordon, *Interactions of Nutrition and Infection* (World Health Organization, Geneva, 1968).

10. Management Sciences for Health, *A Field Survey.*

11. Management Sciences for Health, *Initial Analysis and Work Plan, Management Support for Rural and Family Health Services* (Cambridge, Mass.: MSH, 1974).

12. Gordon C. Whiting and Rufus B. Hughes, *The Afghan Farmer: A Report of a Survey* (Robert Nathan Associates, Washington, D.C., 1972).

13. Carl E. Taylor, et al., *Interactions between Health and Population* (Studies in Family Planning, The Population Council, New York, 1976).

14. Everett M. Rogers, *The Communication of Innovation* (Glencoe: Free Press, 1971).

Appendix B:
The Indigenous Rural
Health System

A. Health-Seeking Opportunities and Agencies of Care

When considering alternatives for expanding health care to remote rural areas, the role of the traditional health system and that of the indigenous practitioners had to be closely examined. In Afghan villages there are a number of different health-care treatment possibilities open to villagers. An overview of the rural health-care system is given in Figure B–1.

The Home

The single most common source of health care in rural Afghanistan is undoubtedly the household. It is not surprising that the Afghan household, which strives for self-sufficiency in most of its other essential needs, would have the capability of caring for many of its health needs within the walls of its compound. Treatments that are carried out entirely or partially within the home include the following.

Bed Rest: Sick individuals are expected to rest. When possible, their household responsibilities are taken over by others and their health needs are attended to by family members, most frequently older women.

Prayer and Vows: One of the first actions mentioned for treating illness is prayer. Often the prayers take on the form of a vow: "If my son is allowed to live, I will visit the shrine every Friday for a year."

Diet: There are many dietary prescriptions associated with the treatment of an illness. The predominant concept of diet during illness follows the Greek humoral beliefs of hots and colds. The diet of each individual is determined according to the body temperature of an individual as well as the perceived hot or cold nature of his or her illness. Foods and medicines are likewise

---

Existing health beliefs, practices, and pathways to care formed the ground on which all program activities were conducted. In Afghanistan, appreciation of these factors came from colleagues, earlier studies, field experience, and surveys conducted for the purpose of developing the understanding necessary for appropriate contribution to rural health work. This appendix summarizes some of these factors, and examines the health system from the village perspective, a useful strategy suggested to the team by Byron and Mary Jo Good.

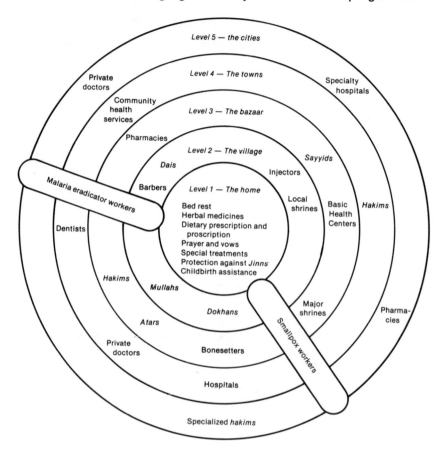

Figure B-1. Overview of Afghan Rural Health System

classified as to their "temperature" and the proper alignment of body temperature and food temperature is strived for.

Herbal Medicine: Herbal medicines play an important role in home treatment. There is a known herbal treatment for almost every set of signs and symptoms. These medicines, usually readily available within the vicinity of the household, but also purchased from herbal shopkeepers or *atars* at the bazaar, are usually the domain of the older women of the household.

Special Treatments: There are a number of special treatments whose origin is the home. One example is the special treatment for fevers and injuries in which a patients is wrapped in goat skins (*post-i-gosphand*). Another example is the practice of caring for a weak and thin child by gathering wheat from seven different households in the village and baking it into a bread to be shared by at least forty women. Many other treatments such as treatment of wounds, skin infections, eyes, and aches and pains also take place in the home.

Childbirth: Pregnancy and childbirth are recognized as times of exceptional physical and emotional problems for women. While many women make use of the *dai*, or traditional midwife, approximately half of all women report receiving childbirth assistance from other women in their household.

Protection Against Jinns: *Jinns* (evil spirits) represent a very serious threat to the health of young children. As might be expected, there is a series of rituals and protective actions to help guard an individual, especially a newborn against these evil spirits. One example is the use of an amulet, or *tawiz,* which is an inscription from the Koran sewn into cloth and worn around the child's neck from birth. Another preventive measure is the *shewest,* whereby a child drinks water into which a *mullah* has immersed paper on which he has written the verses of the Koran.

The home is the source of first resort for most illnesses. The health activities at this level are most frequently the responsibilities of women, with men, as one example, having only limited knowledge of such information as the best herbs to use for an illness. Men are explicitly proscribed from active participation in childbirth, other than for such activities as the transport of women to the doctor or a hospital in the event of a complication.

The treatments administered at home share the characteristics of being traditional in nature and inexpensive. They are the first line of defense against illness. If they fail to prove effective, a decision must be made as to the next level of care that will be sought. This is a decision that involves the potential expenditure of money and the arrangement of transportation. At this point, decisions about care become a matter for the attention of men in the household. Depending on the nature of the illness, the attitudes of the men, and the amount of money available to the family, care may be sought from any one of the following levels or, as commonly occurs, from several at once.

The Village

In the village, there are frequently people who can be turned to in the event of a health problem. These include the following.

Dais: In many villages, there are women specialized in childbirth who come to a woman's home at the time of birth. While the skills and qualifications are usually varied, *dais* are often older women who have raised their own families and who have turned to midwifery as a means of supplementing a meager income. *Dais* often visit a woman in advance of delivery to examine her, and after birth, they will continue to visit the home to observe the condition of mother and child, offer advice, and frequently to assist with household chores.

Barbers: There are a number of services, in addition to cutting hair and shaving, provided by the village barber. Barbers perform circumcisions, pull teeth, and draw blood to release the "bad blood" considered to be the cause of many illnesses. There are many indications that the barber's role as bleeder is one that is diminishing. Blood letting is frequently described by villagers as something "done in the past, but not anymore." The fact that only 6.8 percent of respondents in the three-province survey (1976–1977) reported having used the barber's service in the last year supports this notion.

The *Mullah:* In each village there is found one or more religious leaders who in addition to leading the community in prayer and interpreting the Holy Koran in the context of everyday village life plays an important role in curing and preventing illness. One of the main services of the *mullah* is the preparation of the *tawiz,* which is an amulet consisting of appropriate verses of the Holy Koran that is worn around a patient's neck or pinned to his clothes. The *tawiz* can be both curative, as with adults, or preventative, as can be seen in its use in preventing *jinns* in children. The *mullah* is said to have his greatest effectiveness in treating emotional problems, nervousness, anxiety, mental illness, and illnesses due to evil spirits. He also may play an important role in filtering illnesses and making appropriate referrals to health services outside the village.

One reflection of the importance of the *mullah*'s role in health is that 48 percent of households reported having used his services in the prior year, with an average of 3.2 visits per household.

Dokhandars: Dokhandars are village shopkeepers selling a variety of essential items, frequently including medicines such as aspirin, vitamin C., Vicks Vaporub, and other preparations. They appear not to sell antibiotics or other prescription drugs. They also appear to play only a very limited role in providing service and are not viewed favorably by villagers as a source of care. Their potential lies in use as a more structured means of distributing medications.   .

Injectionists: As was mentioned in appendix A, many villagers report knowing someone in their own village who could give them an injection if required. These injectionists most often assist in administering medicines the villagers have received from physicians, but some injectionists have been reported to purchase their own supplies of drugs. Twenty-eight percent of households reportedly have used an injectionist in the previous year, demonstrating their importance to the village and supporting the argument that injectionists should be screened for their appropriateness for training as village health workers.

Local Shrines: Almost every village has a shrine, usually the burial place of an exceptionally pious ancestor, that is venerated and called upon for its ability to cure illnesses and bring about favors.

Although there are a number of important health services that are carried out at the village level, they tend to be of a relatively unspecialized nature, provided by part-time practitioners. More specialized services are encountered at the level of the bazaar.

The Bazaar: A large bazaar or marketplace supplies a number of villages with the goods and services they require. Here the specialist, be he gunsmith or pharmacist, can establish his trade and draw on a large enough population to earn a livelihood. At this level can be found both traditional and modern health practitioners, including the following.

Pharmacists: There is no modern health service that reaches as deeply or pervasively into rural Afghanistan as the pharmacy. There are at least 500 in the country, with at least one in every major market settlement. They stock and sell a large variety of both prescription and nonprescription drugs. There can be little doubt that the compounder in the pharmacy is an important primary health-care provider, especially in areas where there is no doctor. Not only does he provide advice to his customers, but he may administer injections as well. An indication of the importance of the pharmacy is that 60 percent of all households surveyed had used a pharmacy in the prior year, expending 37 percent of their total health budget.

Hakimji: Traditional medical practitioners, or *hakimji,* are found in bazaars, with the more successful ones being located in the cities. These practitioners, often Hindus, use procedures and medicines that descend from the Unani medical traditions of India as well as those from the Greco-Arabic traditions of the West. The influence of the *hakimji* may be on the wane, especially in those areas where they are in natural competition with a physician. Only 10 percent of households reported using the services of a *hakimji,* suggesting that their impact is limited.

Atars: *Atars* are shopkeepers or sidewalk vendors who specialize in the sale of herbal medicines. They are often small-scale operators with little personal knowledge of health and illness. Since many of the herbal medicines used by villagers are well-known plants found growing in their own vicinities, the *atar*'s role is a marginal one, as can be seen by the fact that only 1 percent of the average annual health budget of rural Afghans is expended at the *atar*'s.

Bonesetters: The *shekesta bande,* or bonesetter, is one of the more specialized practitioners. As the name implies, he sets bones. However, he also treats sprains, dislocations, and assorted body pains. The relatively low percentage of households (6 percent) reporting having used the bonesetters in the previous year underestimates his importance. Most Afghans would prefer to go to the bonesetter for a broken bone than to a physician. This preference is apparently empirically derived.

Bonesetting is a profession apparently not so much chosen as thrust upon a person out of the necessity for someone in a community to meet a need for bone repair. Consistent with their working out of demand rather than for economic gain, bonesetters claim not to charge for their services, accepting money only as offered.

Major Shrines: Another source of help lying outside the village is the major shrine, or *ziarat.* Often a *ziarat* will possess renown for its ability to effect a cure for a particular illness, such as rabies, snake bites, deafness, or infertility. One fourth of all households reported use of a *ziarat* in the preceding year.

Not all of the services just described are to be found in each bazaar, and additionally, many village-type practitioners such as barbers, *dais,* injectionists, and *dokhandars* also can be found in large market places.

Towns

In many ways, Afghan towns can be looked upon as enlarged bazaar areas. As such, they contain many of the same services as can be found in the bazaar, but they also may have the following.

Private Doctors: Most towns are large enough to support at least one general physician. Town doctors, like most other doctors in Afghanistan, are usually government-salaried physicians who augment their official practices with private patients seen after official working hours. More than twice as many households make use of town or regional physicians as use Kabul physicians, a pattern that indicates the useful role of the general town physician.

Dentists: Many towns are large enough to support a dentist. However, since trained dentists are in short supply in the country, demand outweighs supply.

Hospitals: Many towns serve as sites for regional hospitals. As with physicians, regional hospitals are used with greater frequency than those of the capital. While the quality of regional hospitals may not be as good as those in Kabul, the expense is much lower, 327 Afghanis versus 909 Afghanis (from the three-province survey, 1976–1977), and thus regional or town hospitals play an important role, especially at greater distances from Kabul.

Generally, health services in towns are less sophisticated than those in cities, but they are also less expensive and more convenient. The net result is that, for many villagers, the regional hospital and the private physicians of towns represent a major source of care. For more serious illness, either acute emergencies or when all else has failed, a decision is frequently made to bring the patient to Kabul for care.

Cities

Not surprisingly, the cities of Afghanistan, especially Kabul, are centers for specialized health services, including the following.

Hospitals: In addition to general hospitals with a variety of specialty departments, there are several specialized hospitals in Kabul, including maternity, children's, tuberculosis, and eye hospitals.

Private Physicians: There are approximately 500 private physicians in Kabul, many of whom are specialists.

Specialized *Hakimji:* There are a number of specialized *hakimjis* in the cities, several of whom draw patients from throughout the country.

B. Existing Health Expenditures

The two health surveys conducted by the team revealed the startling fact that the mean annual personal-health expenditure in rural Afghanistan was seven times the government expenditure. This meant that 87.5 percent of all money spent on health care in Afghanistan came out of the pockets of impoverished villagers. This represented 7.4 percent of the annual household income of the average Afghan family.

When the pattern of household health expenditure was more closely examined, the importance of drugs became very obvious. The average Afghan spent 37 percent of his health "dollar" on pharmacy drugs, and additional money was spent on traditional herbs and medicine. Villagers willingly spent large amounts of money on drugs. Any Afghan village-based health program that could be supported through the purchase of important drugs by villagers had an excellent chance of being financially self-supporting. This information was crucial to the MOPH's decision to have VHWs work without salaries and instead be supported by the sale of a small number of inexpensive, useful drugs.

C. Rural Perspectives on Alternative Sources of Care

The MOPH's decision to train *dais* marked the first time in Afghanistan that a category of traditional practitioner received official recognition from the government. Also, the fact that *dais* were mostly illiterate women meant that the Afghan government was admitting that such women had worth and value and were capable of learning new skills.

From the point of view of Afghan villagers, the most important healthcare consideration is that someone they trust is available and easily accessible, even if that person is not as fully trained as a doctor or nurse. The *dais* were trusted because of their age, experience, and the fact that they had always lived in their village; VHWs, being chosen by the villagers themselves, were chosen in part because of the trust they enjoyed. The three-province survey (1976) indicated very clearly that villagers wanted a VHW; the very positive subsequent reception by villagers of both *dais* and VHWs has demonstrated the great importance attached to these programs.

Appendix C:
The Financial Analysis

The disparity between plans and performance, even in areas where the Ministry had real interest, is evident in the timing of the financial analyses undertaken to assess the economic feasibility of the national health program. The workplan to test the BHC system and the alternative health-delivery systems was established in the fall of 1974. While cost elements experienced or projected for each of the programs were developed as they evolved, no synthesis of all Ministry commitments was attempted until the fall of 1976. Practical and political imperatives swamped planning theory, and program implementation proceeded largely unencumbered by forecasts of financial feasibility.

In the fall of 1976, with WHO encouragement, the Ministry began a country health programming (CHP) exercise. The CHP methodology provides a formal framework for establishing national health needs and resources and for making choices for application of limited resources to these needs. The underlying task was development of another long-range plan as required by the Ministry of Planning. The Ministry had the team and the budget office concentrate on a subset of these tasks, which was defined as a "financial analysis," to examine costs and outputs of various health activities. Multiple sources were used to assemble cost, output, and coverage data: ministry budgets, expenditure estimates, service statistics, existing survey and project data, and specially collected data from ongoing programs. This information was used to develop both *current-status analyses* and *projections for forward planning.*

A. The Current-Status Analysis

The financial analysis was developed in parallel to the ten programs established by the CHP exercise and the priority groups established by the government health policy: infants, children, pregnant and postpartum women, and the labor force. On an aggregate level, table C-1 relates expenditures in the seven major service programs to the priority-population subgroups served, as well as to their proportion of the population and their mortality experience. The important findings include

---

This appendix consists of excerpts from two exercises exploring relationships between investments in and service outputs from Ministry of Public Health Programs.

Table C-1
Program Expenditures Related to Priority Population Estimates,
1977 Plan

	Infants 0-1 Year	Children 1-14 Years	Pregnant Postpartum Women	Labor Force	Total	Percent
1. Immunization	40%	40%	20%	—	9,660	2
	3,864	3,864	1,932			
2. Tuberculosis/leprosy		26%	10%	64%		
	X	9,549	3,673	23,506	36,728	6
3. Malaria	3.7%	47%	7.1%	42%		
	4,500	57,199	8,641	51,114	121,454	22
4. Water supply	3.7%	47%	7.1%	42%		
	1,852	23,523	3,554	21,021	50,050	9
5. Basic health services	7%	37%	6%	50%		
	7,207	38,096	6,178	51,482	102,963	19
6. Hospitals (B)	7%	21%	10%	62%		
	16,035	48,105	22,907	142,023	229,070	42
Total expenditures	33,458	180,336	46,885	289,146	549,900	
Percentage of total health budget	6%	33%	9%	52%	—	100
Percentage of total mortality	38%	24%	---38%---		—	—
Percentage of total population	3.7%	47%	7.1%	42%	—	—

Note: Figures are in Afghanis × 1,000 (50 Afghanis = $1.00).

1. Only 6 percent of total health expenditure was directed at infants, who are nominally listed in the national plan as the highest-priority target group and who incur 40 percent of total mortality, much of it preventable.
2. Only 1.8 percent of health expenditure was devoted to immunization, including BCG, the service with the highest cost-effectiveness among Ministry programs.
3. Basic Health Services received less than half the operating-budget allocation that hospitals received.

Other findings of relevance to rural health include the following:

1. *Private rural health expenditures and services:* Surveys pointed to substantial private interest in and expenditure for health services. Annual household expenditures approximated 1,000 Afghanis, or 140 Afghanis

Table C-2
Unit Cost-per-Output Comparisons of MOPH Programs and Target Populations

| Program | Output Unit | Target Populations | | | |
		Infants	Children	Pregnant and Postpartum Women	Labor Force
Immunization[a]	Contact	19	19	19	
Tuberculosis/leprosy[b]	Case treated		1050	1050	1050
Malaria[c]	Contact	15	15	15	15
Basic health services[d]	Contact	47	47	47	47
Hospitals[e]	Discharge	1930	1930	990	4000
Water supply[f]	Recipient	31	31	31	31

Note: Figures are in Afghanis per unit output.

[a] Calculated from 1977 immunization 7-year plan.

[b] Calculated from 1977 tuberculosis 7-year plan.

[c] Calculated from 1977 Malaria Institute 7-year plan.

[d] Calculated from 1977 BHS estimated expenditure.

[e] Management Sciences for Health, *Financial Analysis of Health Programs* (Cambridge, Mass.: 1977)

[f] Calculated from 1977 water supply 7-year plan.

per person, which is five to seven times the annual per capita budget of the Ministry. Villagers both within and beyond the reach of Ministry programs seek a wide variety of services.

2. *Comparison of unit cost per output relations for six Ministry programs:* Table C-2 outlines relationships between the costs and units of output as defined by the programs for Basic Health Centers. Improved management and realistic levels of Ministry resources for operation effectively tripled service volume at stable budget levels, producing per visit costs of 47 Afghanis.

The immunization program delivers its service for 19 Afghanis per contact, and along with malaria, it represented the least expensive direct-service program of the Ministry. The tuberculosis program costs more than 1,000 Afghanis per treated case, and hospitalization costs 1,000 to 4,000 Afghanis per discharge. Approximation of program cost per output relations was a useful and controversial step in focusing Ministry attention and priorities, as reflected in their budget investment at the time.

B. Projections for Forward Planning

Ministry departments and the CHP team proceeded to develop individual plans for each program. These were then analyzed jointly to assess potential financial and target-population impact. Successive iterations of alternative plans and funding levels were used by the Ministry in the context of an intense political advocacy process to arrive at the final plan.

Three illustrations of the uses of the financial analysis may be useful:

1. It provided a *simple indicator of relative changes in Ministry priorities.* A comparison of the percentages of total Ministry budget devoted to each program results in the bar graph in figure C-1 which was relatively easy for nonnumerically oriented staff, of which there are many, to understand. This was probably the most frequently used and understood method.

2. It allowed *simulation of alternative investment strategies.* Decisions on hospital expansion and location are complicated by many factors beyond the political; strategies for use and development of related facilities, assumptions for utilization and staffing, availability of investment capital and/or donor interest, construction schedules and commitments to maintenance expenditure are all important examples. Discussion and planning of alternatives was made more tractable by specifying assumptions made for each of these factors and then projecting schedules and financial requirements. While still simplified, this level of detailed projection taxed many in the planning process who had the responsibility but neither the experience nor the time to work through the methodology. One practical result, however, was a decision to convert small, underutilized hospitals that operated at great expense into health centers.

3. *Assessment of inflation impact and government budget increase ceilings.* In spite of consistent experience with inflation and government ceilings on percentage increases in Ministry budgets, program commitments—particularly for construction and expansion of facilities— tended to be made independently of realistic assessment of the feasibility of financial support or staffing. A second phase of the financial analysis was used to point out and demonstrate two points:

   a. That the CHP plan would require hospitals and basic health services alone to absorb virtually the entire Ministry budget for operating expenses over the ensuing 7 years.

   b. That alternative combinations of program expansion, realignment of priorities, and utilization of the existing high levels of personal health expenditure presented more realistic approaches to health-program goals.

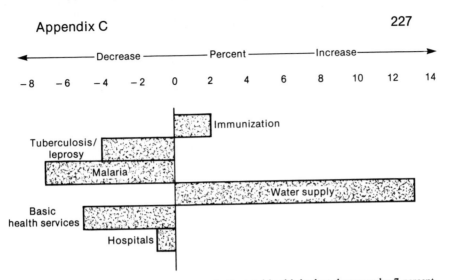

Example: The share of the malaria program in the total health budget decreases by 7 percent from 1356-1361.

Figure C-1. Changing MOPH *Priorities, 1356-1361* (1977-1982) (as indicated by changes in the percent of the total health budget allocated to the service programs)

In sum, the first steps toward financial planning did make simple and important improvements in the Ministry planning process. However, planning remained an exercise that was largely divorced from the actual operation of the Ministry. These observations on the process should be viewed in that light.

Appendix D: Basic Health Services in Developing Countries: A Model and a Critique

John W. LeSar

A. The Jobs of a BHS System

A health system has two main jobs: (1) to provide relief from fear, pain, and suffering for people who are sick or injured, and (2) to reduce mortality, morbidity, and disability in the population. The first job is to provide relief from fear, pain, and suffering. When people are sick or injured, they seek help, and the health system must, to the best of its ability, provide that help. These services are *demanded* by the people, and medical relief is their number one health priority. The performance of the health system in providing relief to sick or injured people is the criterion on which the people judge the success of the health system. These services are to individuals and are generally curative medicinal services.

The second job of the health system is to reduce mortality, morbidity, and disability in the population. On an individual basis, curative medicine performs this job through proper diagnosis and treatment of sick or injured people. However, reductions in mortality, morbidity, and disability in developing countries are best achieved by studying, in the population, the epidemiology of disease and its direct and contributing causes. The disease causes are often easy for health professionals to understand, but are beyond the knowledge of most other people. For this reason, people do not demand public-health programs—professionals promote them. Thus planned public-health programs must convince the population (or force, as seen in certain totalitarian regimes) to try new things. This change process in the population is not easy to achieve and requires a managed approach.

These two jobs, when implemented through a large government system, require extensive management and technical support. These support systems have their own objectives, but must always serve the two jobs of the health system: medical relief and reductions in mortality and morbidity through individual services and community-based public-health programs.

The team's experience with Basic Health Centers in Afghanistan is discussed in chapter 2. Out of that experience come some impressions about what basic health services, often unrealistically, are expected to provide. Jack LeSar here presents one view of the implications underlying commonly held expectations for Basic Health Centers.

Historically, health planners have tried to do these jobs in two main ways in rural areas. The first job of providing medical relief has been mostly tried through establishing a wide network of service-delivery units in rural areas often called Basic Health Centers (BHCs). These BHCs are staffed by doctors and paramedical (middle-level) workers, and they are supported by small hospitals at the district or province level.

To reduce mortality, morbidity, and disability in the population, both BHCs and specially managed public-health programs have been used. The BHCs obviously try to reduce mortality, morbidity, and disability in individuals who visit the facility by correct diagnosis and treatment for illness or injury. They also try to prevent mortality, morbidity, and disability for special target groups such as pregnant women, young children, and tuberculosis patients who visit the facility. In addition, BHCs in many countries have been given responsibilities in implementing public-health programs for the population living near the BHC. BHCs have a dismal record in carrying out these community-based public-health activities. The specially managed public-health programs (often called "vertical programs" because they are managed by special units) have a much better record in influencing mortality and morbidity for the special conditions they attempt to ameliorate. Smallpox eradication is the most successful example. Other specially managed programs have been less successful, but, *compared with the Basic Health Center approach,* are much more successful in carrying out community-based public-health programs.

Thus the BHC traditionally has two components: services to individuals at the BHC itself and services to community groups as a public-health service unit. In other words, the BHC, the most peripheral unit of the health system, is an *integrated unit* expected to provide individual services and public-health programs. This is a most interesting phenomenon because health systems in developed countries usually separate these components, while health planners in developing countries (often advised by developed-country advisors) have tried to integrate these two activities at the BHC.

Recently, a new approach has received wide publicity in the international health literature and strong promotion (to the point of coercion) by the World Health Organization. This is the "primary health care" movement, which has centered on using the villagers themselves to improve their own health (the now famous maxim "health by the people"). This approach has strong merit because most developing countries cannot provide reasonable access to the Basic Health Center for large numbers of their people, since there is a large "social gap" between the traditional cultures of villagers and the more modern cultural values of professionals and paramedical workers, and because villagers can participate in their own development. This approach has now received some limited application, and experience indicates that the trained villager can provide some selected individual services in the village—both for medical relief and to prevent deaths from some common disease killers (especially diarrhea in young children). However, many health planners are advocating that the village health workers can perform public-health functions as well if supported by BHCs. This is also most interesting, because the Basic Health Center cannot provide a decent public-health function on its own and yet it is expected to provide additional support and guidance for villagers who are being given public-health tasks that are not demanded by the people and are difficult to achieve.

B. A Basic Health Services System and its Functions

Any basic health services system usually has four major components: (1) service-delivery units, (2) management/administrative units, (3) training units, and (4) technical-support units.

The *rural-service delivery units* are those units which actually provide medical/public-health services to the population. In Afghanistan, they are called Basic Health Centers. (Village-based services will be discussed later.) The *management/administrative units* have the job of planning, managing, and evaluating the service-delivery units. In Afghanistan, the main management/administrative unit for Basic Health Centers (BHCs) had been the Basic Health Services Department located in the Ministry of Public Health in Kabul. During the course of the project, other intermediate management/administrative units were attempted, namely, the regional offices. *Training units* provide increased skills to personnel in the system. In Afghanistan, there have been training units within the BHS Department and in other parts of the MOPH. *Technical-support units* are units supplying special services of a technical nature. The main technical units affecting BHSD operations have been the National Laboratory, which trains and supervises laboratory workers who work in BHCs; the Malaria Institute, which supplies malaria microscopists to BHCs; and the Avicenna Pharmaceutical Institute, which produces drug supplies for BHCs as well as other parts of the MOPH.

The intent of the Basic Health Services Project has always been to further develop the basic health services system. Thus the underdevelopment of the system at the beginning of the project is a basic assumption for all further activities. If the basic health services system in Afghanistan was underdeveloped at the beginning of the project (few would argue that it was not), the question arises as to what a developed basic health services system should look like. That is, what would be the services provided by a well-developed BHC? What then would be the management/administrative units to effectively support a well-developed BHC? What then would be the training-support and technical-support functions necessary to have a complete well-developed basic health services system?

The Well-Developed BHC: Its Services and Support Functions

The BHC should offer the following high-quality services to individuals who visit the BHC:

1. *Sickness-care services:* These include diagnosis, treatment, and individual counseling of the sick patient for common medical, surgical, gynecological, physical/orthopedic, and mental problems.
2. *Maternal-care services:* These include all aspects of pregnancy care/ prenatal care, labor and delivery, and postpartum care. In addition, usually family planning and care during lactation are included in maternal-care services. A women who is sick but not pregnant would be included in the sickness-care classification.
3. *Child-care services:* These include all aspects of well-child care: assessment of growth and development (nutritional services are included here), immunizations against childhood diseases, and vision and hearing testing for older children.
4. *Food-distribution services:* These include distribution of dried milk powder, oil, and wheat through the World Food Distribution program to high-risk pregnant mothers and high-risk young children.

The well-developed BHC should offer the following high-quality *public-health programs* to communities:

1. *Communicable-disease and high-risk surveillance program:* This includes surveillance of the entire population at least three times a year for tuberculosis, trachoma, childhood malnutrition, high-risk pregnancy, family-planning motivation, births, and deaths.
2. *Community-immunization program:* This includes immunization of at least 75 percent of the entire susceptible community against smallpox, diphtheria, tetanus, whooping cough, tuberculosis, measles, and polio.
3. *Special-care follow-up program:* This includes frequent follow-up of selected families who have communicable diseases or high-risk children or mothers (tuberculosis, about once a month; childhood malnutrition, moderate, about once a month, severe, weekly; active trachoma, every 2 weeks).

4. *Family-planning motivation program:* This includes quarterly visits to all households.
5. *School health program:* This includes quarterly vision and hearing testing.
6. *Safe-water program:* This calls for safe water at the time of use for 80 percent of households based on a filter system (safe source) and a health-education program (safe storage and use).
7. *Safe-latrine and safe-waste-disposal program:* This calls for water-seal latrines or covered-pit latrines that are maintained effectively in 80 percent of households; that is, that 80 percent of households dispose of wastes adequately.
8. *Public facilities inspection programs:* This calls for quarterly inspection of all restaurants, hotels, and other public facilities likely to promote disease.
9. *Health-education programs:* These include twice yearly group sessions to all public organized groups, and more frequently to target groups (mothers' clubs especially).

Table D-1 summarizes these functions and their locations.

*Staffing Patterns Necessary to Adequately Implement the
Medical Public-Health Functions*

If the BHC is to truly serve a population of 25,000 people with individual services at the BHC and community-based public-health programs, it must have adequate numbers of staff. Given the services discussed previously, the following staffing patterns would be necessary to effectively implement the jobs given to the BHC.

Individual Services at the BHC Itself: Individual services at the BHC are given when demanded by the population. Therefore, the number of personnel needed is determined by the number of visitors per day. WHO has recommended an average of 2.5 visits per person per year as a desirable standard. For the well-developed BHC in this example, 1.5 visits per person per year will be used as a *minimum standard.* That is, if the BHC does not see $1.5 \times 25,000$ persons per year, it is not providing the minimum number of individual services at the BHC (in developed countries, the average visits per person per year are well over 3). For our well-developed BHC, the yearly workload for individual services demanded by the people should exceed 37,500, or about 150 visits per day, not including food distribution.

Table D-1
Service Locations of Well-Developed BHCs

Program	Components	Location of Services	
		At BHC Itself	In Community
Sickness care	Medical	X	
	Surgical/dressing	X	
	Physical/orthopedic	X	None
	Gynecological	X	
	Mental	X	
Maternal care	Prenatal care	X	Surveillance program
	Labor and delivery	X	On request
	Postpartum	X	No
	Family planning	X	Family-planning motivation program
	Care during lactation	X	No
Child care	Growth and development	X	Surveillance program
	Immunizations	X	Community immunization program
	School eye and hearing testing		School health program
Communicable disease control	Malaria smears	X	Surveillance program
	Tuberculosis smears	X	No
	Malaria surveillance		Surveillance program
	Tuberculosis surveillance and defaulter control		Special-care program
	Trachoma		Surveillance program
	Immunizations		Community immunization program
Environmental health	Safe water		Safe-water program
	Safe latrine		Safe-latrine program
	Waste disposal		Waste-disposal program
	Public facilities inspection		Inspection program
Health education	To patients	X	
	To groups at BHC	X	
	To schools		School health program
	To community groups		Health-education program
Food distribution	Children	X	None
	Women	X	

The distribution of these visits should be as follows:

	Visits	Percentage
Sickness care	112	75
Maternal care	9	6
Well-child care	29	19
Total	150	100

These numbers were derived as follows: if one assumes a crude birth rate (CBR) of 43 per 1000, then there are 1075 pregnant women in a population of 25,000 during a given year. If the average woman makes only 2 prenatal visits, and if there are 250 working days per year in a BHC, then there would be 9 maternal-care visits per day. Given these assumptions there would be 950 children 0–11 months in the population. If each visits the BHC 4 times per year (with 3 of these visits for immunization), and if the 1750 children aged 12–35 months each make 2 visits per year to the BHC, then there would be 7300 annual well-child care visits or 29 visits per day.

Three BHC personnel are primarily responsible for providing the individual services to people who come to the BHC. These are the doctor, the female health worker (nurse-midwife or auxiliary nurse-midwife), and the male nurse. The doctor offers services to sick people and sees referrals from the female worker or male nurse. The female worker sees sick children and some sick adult women and deals with routine maternal and well-child care. The male nurse offers individual services to sick people mainly for minor surgical and dressing care. Given the assumptions that the doctor sees 60 percent of sickness care, 10 percent of maternal and child care (referrals), 5 percent of male-nurse patients, and spends 10 minutes per patient: $(112 \times .6) \times (38 \times .1) \times (112 \times .1 \times .05)$ = 72 patients × 10 minutes/patient ÷ 60 minutes/hour = 11.8 hours; the female worker sees 30 percent of sickness care, and all maternal and well child care at 10 minutes/person, and the male sees 10 percent of sickness care at 30 minutes/person, then the workload for each of these personnel at a well-developed BHC would be as follows:

Worker	Patients per Day	Time Required per Day	Workers Required to Fulfill This Obligation
Doctor	72	12 hours	2
Female worker	72	12 hours	2
Male nurse	11	6 hours	1

One other individual service regularly given at the BHC is food distribution. If one assumes that one-half of the people visiting the BHC for maternal care and child care would be eligible, then there would be nineteen visits per day for food distribution. In a well-developed BHC, this function would be filled by an administrative clerk. If it takes 2 hours per day to prepare the food-distribution requirements and 10 minutes per recipient, the manpower needed would be as follows:

Worker	Clients per Day	Time Required per Day	Workers Required to Fulfill This Function
Clerk	19	5 hours	1

Public-Health Programs in the Community: Community health programs are planned programs. In a well-developed BHC, each program must have sufficient personnel to do the job at some minimum level of performance. Therefore, it is important to analyze each program to see what the manpower requirements are.

The communicable disease and high-risk surveillance program has as its objectives the visiting of each household in the community at least four times a year. The surveillance itself can be done by trained villagers. The number of villagers needed is determined by workload analysis. Assuming that each villager can visit eight households a day and that about 3,675 households exist in the population (6.8 persons per household in Afghanistan), then one surveillance worker could visit 440 households in each quarter of the year (8 households per day × 55 working days in one quarter = 440 households). The number of workers needed, then, is 3,675 ÷ 440 = 8 to 9 workers. This is the number of workers needed to provide surveillance services to the community.

The community-immunization program has as its objective the immunization of 75 percent of susceptibles in the community. Therefore, the workload is dependent on the number of susceptibles. Assuming that all persons are susceptible, then the workload is 75 percent × 25,000 = 18,500. In a well-developed BHC, the worker should be able to visit about sixteen households per day. If each household requries three visits to complete the immunization services, then each worker can cover 1,200 households per year (16 × 5 days × 15 weeks). Therefore, in the first year, three vaccinators would be required. After the first year, all households should be visited once a year to find children born in the last year but whose mothers have not brought them to the well-child program at the BHC (where they receive immunizations) and to find new families in the community. Therefore, one or two vaccinators would be sufficient.

The special-care follow-up program would give special attention to high-risk families. In Afghanistan, about 20 percent of the 3,675 households would be high-risk requiring monthly visits or about 8,820 total visits per year. One worker could visit about six households per day during the 250 working days of the year, so six special-care follow-up workers would be needed. These workers should be middle-level female health workers.

The family-planning motivation program has as its objective quarterly visits to all households. This activity can be done by the surveillance workers as they make quarterly visits. However, interested families should receive follow-up by other family-planning workers; therefore 735 households should have a follow-up visit. If a middle-level family-planning motivator visits four households per day, then one middle-level family planning motivator is needed to supplement the surveillance workers.

The school health program offers vision and hearing tests to the school plus surveillance for selected infectious diseases (school health teaching is the responsibility of the teacher and not the BHC). Each school should be visited quarterly, and each visit should take one day. In a population of 25,000, there will be about 6,925 children in the 5 to 14 age group. If one half of them are in school, there will be about 3,462 school children in three to six schools. Thus the workload is five schools per quarter, or 1 week of work per quarter, requiring about one-tenth of one female worker's time.

The safe-water program has an objective of 80 percent of households having safe water at the time of use. This would require safe sources of water plus safe storage and use of water. The number of households to be included would be 2,940. If the entire population were densely crowded, perhaps a few water sources would be sufficient. More likely, in Afghanistan, for example, at least 150 safe sources would be needed (tube wells).

Each source would require construction, but let us assume that a construction department did that work. Each source would require two kinds of maintenance: preventive maintenance and repairs of broken-down sources. Data on repair rates are hard to find, but for the purpose of this analysis, let us assume that 5 percent of all tube wells need repair each month and that two wells can be repaired by one person in one day. In that case, about eight wells would need to be repaired each month, or 4 work days per month for one worker. In addition, a good safe-water program would have preventive maintenance, where all sources would receive monthly visits. If there are 150 sources and the worker can visit 10 each day, then 15 days per month would be required to serve a community of 25,000 people.

However, for an effective safe-water program, having safe sources is not enough. It is also necessary to have safe storage and safe use of the water. This requires a community health-education program in which each household is investigated and those households not practicing water safety receive health education. In Afghanistan, one could assume that 75 percent of households do not practice water safety in storage and use. These households would require quarterly visits by safe-water-program personnel to have some reasonable effect. These habits are difficult to change and would require about 30-minute to 1-hour health-education sessions. One worker could do about six of these in one day. Based on 75 percent of 3,675 households, an effective safe-water program would require two workers to give safe-water education. The safe-water program would then require three persons to do an adequate job.

A safe-latrine and waste-disposal program might have as its objectives 80 percent of households having safe latrines and safe waste disposal. This would require construction, which would probably be a BHC function. Construction of safe pit latrines would require 1 day per household. In addition, this would require maintenance of latrine and waste-disposal safety through inspection programs for those households in which latrines are not well maintained and wastes are poorly disposed of. If the construction program had an objective of helping install 25 percent of households per year with pit latrines, then 735 working days would be required. This would mean three permanent latrine-construction advisors would be needed. The latrine-maintenance program would be similar to the safe-water education program and would require two workers. Therefore, the safe-latrine and waste-disposal program would require five workers in a well-developed BHC.

The public-facilities inspection program has an objective of inspecting all restaurants, hotels, and selected public facilities quarterly. In a community of 25,000, the number would be variable, but probably would include at least twenty facilities of varying sizes. Each inspection could take 1 hour, and therefore, about six could be done in any one day. Thus this activity would take about 3 days per quarter, or 12 days per year. This would be about 5 percent of another worker's time.

The health-education program has an objective of providing twice-yearly health education to groups in the community, with special emphasis on maternal health and childrearing. If each ten households were considered to be one group (fifteen women—about the maximum size of groups where discussion and question and answer periods are effective), then about 736 group sessions should be given in one year. A health educator could give about two of these in one day in the community, and thus, 368 working days would be required to fulfill this function. In addition, group health education should be given daily at the BHC as a full-time job. Thus, an effective health education program would require about three workers.

When one adds up the staffing required to adequately provide each of the BHC functions—individual services and community public-health programs—the results shown in table D–2 are seen. This table shows that about thirty-five workers would be necessary just to provide the medical/public-health services to a community of 25,000 people. While this may seem excessive, one should consider how many such workers would exist to serve a community of 25,000 people in a developed country—probably over 280. (For example, in the United States, there would be 17 to 20 doctors, 70 to 80 nurses, 70 to 80 other paramedical personnel, and probably over 100 public health workers working in various areas including the water and sewer departments. The total is about 280 persons.)

Medical/Public-Health Skills Needed in a Well-Developed
BHC to Adequately Carry Out Its Functions

Having a sufficient number of service personnel is hardly adequate to effectively carry out the functions a well-developed BHC would have to perform.

Table D-2
Staffing Required for BHC Functions

Individual services	Worker Type	Number Required
	Doctor	2
	Female worker	2
	Male nurse	1
	Food distribution clerk	1
Community public-health programs		
Surveillance	Trained villagers	9
Immunization	Vaccinator	2
Special care	Female health worker	6
Family planning	Female middle-level motivator	1
School health	Female health worker	1/10
Safe water	Well maintenance	1
	Well inspection and water education	2
Safe latrine	Latrine construction	3
	Inspection and education	2
Public-facilities inspection	Inspector/health educator	1/20
Health education	Health educators	3
		35 +
	Total workers for medical/ public-health services, say	35

Each worker needs the proper skills to do his or her job. Table D-3 shows what overall skills would be necessary in each worker to effectively do the job. Of importance is the fact that the BHC is a unit that offers outpatient individual services in a rural setting. It is not an urban hospital with bed patients. In the community public-health areas, the same holds true. The BHC is a rural public health unit, and workers need skills in working in public-health programs in the rural environment, not in working in the capital city or other large urban areas. This table demonstrates that advanced skills are needed by most workers to perform their jobs. Without these skills, workers are unlikely to be able to work effectively. When this happens, morale falls and the BHC does not do its job.

These skill needs demonstrate the importance of the training function. Workers must have specific training in the environment in which they will work, and they must perform their jobs under the supervision of their teachers until they can do them without supervision. Each job must have a careful analysis of its component parts, and the training organization must ensure that workers have all the skills necessary for each and every part of their jobs. Training in urban environments and hospital settings is inadequate preparation for work in a well-developed BHC.

Table D–3
Overall Skills Necessary in BHC Personnel

Worker Type	Jobs	Skills Needed to Perform Effectively
Doctor	Sickness care	Outpatient medical diagnosis and treatment Outpatient minor surgical procedures Outpatient care for sprains, fractures, contusions, including the ability to put on a cast Outpatient gynecological care and referral care for complications of pregnancy Outpatient mental health care Emergency diagnosis and treatment for life-threatening conditions
Female workers (ANM or midwife)	Sickness care	Outpatient diagnosis and treatment for common minor medical conditions of women and young children
	Maternal care at the BHC	Outpatient care for routine pregnancies, diagnosis of high-risk pregnancies, management of labor and delivery for normal pregnancies, routine postpartum care, and care during lactation
	Child care at the BHC	Outpatient care for children who are not acutely sick, including assessment of growth and development, assessment of the need for immunizations, and vision and hearing testing
	Special care follow-up in the the community	Follow-up through home visiting of high-risk pregnancies and high-risk children, particularly malnourished children
Male nurse	Sickness care at the BHC	Outpatient care for trauma and burns
Food-distribution clerk	Food distribution at the BHC	Reading, writing, clerical recording and reporting, filing of records, preparation of WFP materials
Village-surveillance workers	Surveillance program in the community	Reading of surveillance forms (may be nonliterate forms), ability to walk in the community and talk to people, basic knowledge of diseases and conditions under surveillance, basic communications skills

Table D–3 (continued)

Vaccinator	Vaccination at the BHC community immunization program	Storage and care of vaccines, refrigerator maintenance, injection techniques, basic recording, and filing
Family planning motivator	Motivation in the community for interested couples	Advanced motivational skills and communication skills
Well-maintenance specialist	Safe-water program	Repair of tube wells, ordering and storage of parts and lubricants, preventive maintenance of tube wells
Water-safety educator	Safe-water program	Advanced water-safety education and communication skills
Latrine-construction specialists	Safe-latrine and waste-disposal program	Construction of pit and water-seal latrines, ordering, storing, and maintenance of equipment
Latrine and waste-disposal safety specialist	Safe-latrine and waste-disposal program	Advanced communication skills, advanced latrine and waste-disposal maintenance skills
Health-education specialists (MCH)	Community health-education program	Advanced subject matter and communications skills, community organization and group dynamics skills

C. Management/Administrative Functions of Well-Developed BHCs

Although the BHC is primarily a service-delivery unit, it has many management/administrative functions as well. It has *internal management* functions to manage its own personnel. In a well-developed BHC, there would be about thirty-five service workers providing individual services at the BHC and working in nine community public-health programs. Since individual services at the BHC are given on demand to people who visit the BHC, the internal management of this function of the BHC is not too difficult. However, the community public-health programs are planned activities and require sufficient personnel and skilled personnel if these programs are to have effective management/administrative support. The BHC also exists as part of a larger system and thus has various *recording and reporting functions* for higher-level management units. Table D–4 lists the major management/administrative support functions necessary to operate a well-developed BHC.

This table demonstrates the many management/administrative tasks in operating the BHC and its programs, particularly the community public-health programs. In a well-developed BHC, what would be the staffing patterns necessary to give adequate management/administrative support to BHC medical/public-health services and programs?

Staffing Patterns for Management/Administrative Personnel in a Well-Developed BHC

Table D–5 lists the staffing needs of a well-developed BHC for management/administrative functions. For the support staff, only the administrator is shown, although there would be clerks, drivers, sweepers, and so forth in addition. The table shows that an additional eight management personnel would be needed, including one community public-health program manager and five supervisors for the community health programs with three or more personnel.

Management/Administrative Skills Needed in a Well-Developed BHC

Table D–5 shows that the doctor and the pharmacist have management/administrative functions in addition to their medical/public-health job (doctor) or their technical-support job (pharmacist). The other eight jobs are purely management jobs. The skills needed for these jobs are shown in table D–6.

The management/administrative responsibilities of the doctor are limited if there is a community public-health program manager to manage all public-health activities. If the doctor remains in charge of this well-developed BHC, then the doctor must have necessary skills in public-health subject matter to give effective guidance to the community public-health program.

In this approach to the management of a well-developed BHC, the doctor retains a primary focus on sickness care and the quality of maternal and child care in the BHC. Since he has spent about 6 to 8 years preparing for this job, he should be able to perform this work effectively. The doctor would require specific training in performance evaluation, communications, on-the-job training, and motivational methods to supplement his usual medical education, and he should have adequate training in medical school in public-health conditions of his country.

The key to the success of the community-health activities is the community-health program manager. This person should be skilled in public-health content and basic management. Either a college-degree program in public-health management or a 2-year special course would provide such a worker with the critical management skills so lacking throughout the developing world.

Table D–4
Management/Administrative Functions of Well-Developed BHCs

Function	Necessary components	Activities Needing Function
Planning	Demonstration of need Development of receptive environment Design of the activities and how to do them Design of the management-support systems Manning of the system Field-testing and revisions Start-up planning	The actual planning of BHC activities is the job of the Basic Health Services Department as part of its research-and-development functions. The activities needing planning include the individual services activities, all the public health programs, (surveillance, immunization, special care, family planning, school health, safe water, safe latrine and waste disposal, public-facilities inspection, and health education), and the reporting to higher management units
Operations management	Start-up management	Responsibility of BHS headquarters
	Scheduling of services and workers	Scheduling of individual services and workers
		Scheduling of community public-health programs and workers
		Allocating work among workers
		Maintaining flow of patients through the BHC
	Managing use of supplies and equipment	Ordering and maintaining inventory control for drugs and equipment
	Controlling the quality of of work	Supervising work of individual services activities
		Supervising work of community public-health programs
		Supervising reporting to higher units
	Managing the support systems	Managing the local budget
		Managing holidays and personal leaves
		In-service training
		Maintaining relations with government officials and other decision makers
	Revising and updating the system as new information becomes available	Responsibility of BHS headquarters
Evaluation	Assessing the results of the activities against the plan	Responsibility of BHS headquarters

Besides a community-health program manager, middle-level supervisors are needed to supervise all aspects of the community-health program. For effective programming, an adequate span of control and middle-level supervisory skills must be present so that both diagnostic and corrective-action systems can be developed.

The administrator is another key element in operating effective BHCs. He maintains control over management-support systems, particularly financial control, personnel management, and care of the BHC building and equipment. If these personnel are present, adequately skilled, have adequate budgets, and are adequately supported by higher-level units, the BHC can be an effective force in reducing the mortality, morbidity, and disability of its community of 25,000.

D. Management/Administrative Functions of a
Well-Developed Basic Health Services Headquarters

A basic health services headquarters (BHSHQ) has six main jobs:

1. Management of existing basic health service units and their activities and programs
2. Research and development of new services and programs and research and development to improve existing services and programs.
3. Coordination with other units of government in areas pertaining to basic health services.
4. Training of personnel within the basic health services to maintain and enhance skills.
5. Evaluation of BHS activities/programs.
6. Management of BHSHQ itself and other intermediate management units.

Each of these jobs requires the application of the management process—planning, operations management, and evaluation. Table D-7 shows the activities needing these functions in the area of basic health services in a well-developed BHSHQ.

Staffing Patterns Necessary to Effectively Manage a BHS
System

Within the BHSHQ, there should be smaller units to fulfill the major jobs of the BHSHQ: management of BHCs, research and development of new activities/programs, coordination with other government units, training, evaluation, and headquarters administration. Each of these will be discussed in some detail.

Table D-5
Staffing Needs at a Well-Developed BHC: Managment/Administrative Functions

Function	Individual Services	Community Public-Health Programs
Scheduling	Doctor	Community Health program
Managing use of supplies and equipment	Pharmacists (drug) Logistics specialist (shared)	Logistics specialist (shared)
Controlling the quality of work	Doctor	Surveillance program supervisor
		Special-care program supervisor
		Safe-water program supervisor
		Safe-latrine and waste-disposal supervisor
		Health-education supervisor
Managing the support systems	Administrator (for entire BHC)	

Table D-6
Management/Administrative Jobs in a Well-Developed BHC

Worker Type	Jobs	Skills Needed to Perform Effectively
Doctor	Scheduling	Planning individual services targets
		Planning hours of operation for individual services
		Allocating work among staff for individual services programs
	Quality control for individual services programs	Performance-evaluation skills for medical-care activities, basic teaching and communications skills, motivational skills
Community health program	Overall management of community public health programs	Public-health subject matter, basic planning skills, advanced operations-management skills (all aspects), evaluation skills
Logistics specialists	Managing use of supplies and equipment	Ordering and inventory control for medical and public-health equipment
Program supervisors	Controlling the quality of work	Performance evaluation for public-health activities, basic teaching and communication skills, motivational skills
Administrator	Managing the support systems	Personnel management, financial management, information-system management, physical-plant management

Table D-7

Management/Administrative Functions in a Well-Developed Basic Health Services Headquarters

Function	Necessary Components	Activities Needing Function
Planning	*Existing Programs*	
	Objectives	Individual services activities for BHCs
	Outputs	Community public-health program activities of BHCs
	Quality standards	Coordination planning for logistics, personnel, finance, training
	Inputs	Training activities within BHSHQ
	New Programs	
	Demonstration of need	Research and development of new activities and programs for BHCs
	Development of receptive environment	Research and development of new or improved management/administrative systems
	Design of the services/programs	
	Design of the management support systems	
	Manning of the system	
	Fieldtesting and revisions	
	Start-up planning	
Operations management	Start-up management	New activities or programs of BHCs
		New management/administrative systems within BHCs
	Scheduling of services	Within BHS management/administrative units
		Training activities within BHSHQ
	Managing use of supplies and equipment	Within BHSHQ
		Of BHCs
		Of BHSHQ
	Controlling the quality	Of training within BHSHQ
		Of intermediate management units
	Managing the support systems	Within BHSHQ
	Revising and updating the system as new information becomes available	All BHS units

Table D–7 (continued)

Evaluation	Ensuring the progress toward the objectives	BHC activities and programs
		Workers skills after training

BHC Management Unit: Management of existing activities and programs of BHCs is mainly done through supervision and statistical reports. Effective supervisory control requires a span of control of one supervisor for each five to eight BHCs. A well-developed BHSHQ with 100 BHCs would have from thirteen to twenty supervisory teams. Each team would have one member for supervision of the individual services programs, one member for supervision of each of the major community health programs, one to check supply and equipment maintenance, and one for supervising the support systems. In this situation, there would be eight persons per supervisory team, or from 104 to 160 supervisory personnel. To maintain an adequate span of control of the supervisory teams, three to four supervision managers would be necessary plus one person in charge of the entire supervisory program. Seven to ten clerical personnel would be necessary.

Management of the statistical reporting system would require about one clerk for each twenty BHCs and one manager for statistical reporting, a total of six persons in our example. Thus management of existing BHCs would require about 140 personnel for effective management control exclusive of secretarial help.

Research-and-Development Unit: The research-and-development unit in a well-developed BHSHQ would have one group concentrating on medical/public-health services and another group concentrating on management/administrative functions. Each group probably would have at least five research-and-development personnel. The total would be not less than ten persons.

Coordination Unit: The main jobs for coordination within the ministry involve logistics, personnel, finance, and training. A well-developed BHSHQ would have a management person in each of these areas plus clerical support. In our example, a coordination manager and four management specialists would be adequate plus clerical staff.

Training Unit: The training unit offers in-service training to BHC personnel in medical/public-health skills and in basic management/administrative skills. If each worker is to receive in-service education twice per year for 3 days (once on medical/public-health skills and once in management/administration—a minimal program), with a class size of twenty to thirty, and there are 100 BHCs with eight types of workers in each, then about thirty to forty trainers would be needed. Six to eight trainer supervisors would be needed as well as a training coordinator. In addition, four curriculum developers would be needed and two testing specialists. This curriculum-development and testing unit would require a manager. There also would be a training aids staff of four to eight and a training materials administration staff of ten or more. The whole training unit would require two senior training managers and would have sixty-five or more personnel plus clerical staff.

Evaluation Unit: The evaluation unit would evaluate the activities and programs of existing BHCs and the training unit. It would have specialists for individual-services evaluation and for each of the community public-health program types. In addition, it would have personnel in management-systems evaluation. To support this staff, research-design and statistical personnel would be present as well as an evaluation manager. Most likely, over fifteen persons plus clerical staff would work in such a unit in a system having 100 BHCs.

Headquarters Administration Unit: If the rest of the BHSHQ unit had about 235 personnel plus clerical staff, a headquarters administrative unit would need twenty-five or more people to manage the personnel records, office supplies, pay records, and so forth of such a large system.

This analysis shows that about 260 people plus clerical staff would be necessary to adequately manage a BHS system with 100 BHCs. These people could all be in a BHSHQ, or a BHSHQ plus intermediate management units as an organizational pattern.

Management/Administrative Skills Needed in a
Well-Developed BHS Management System

Table D–8 shows the management/administrative skills needed to optimally manage a well-developed BHS management system. Of importance is that some level of management skills—mostly middle-level and advanced-level skills—is needed to operate a large, decentralized health system effectively.

**E. Planning for the Future: The Nature of the Basic
Health Center**

Afghanistan is not alone in having unrealistic expectations for the Basic Health Center. The generally accepted idea of the BHC, based on the work of John Grant in India in the 1930s and 1940s, has numerous conceptual

Table D–8
**Management/Administrative Skills in a Well-Developed Basic Health
Services Management System: BHC Management Unit**

Worker Type	Jobs	Skills Needed to Perform Effectively	Optimum Qualifications
Supervision program director	Overall management of supervisory program	Advanced management skills with special skills in performance evaluation, worker motivation, training, and communications Advanced medical/public health knowledge	MD/MPH/MBA
Supervision team managers	Direct supervision of five to eight supervisory teams	Same as program director	Same as program director
Individual services supervisors	Supervision of sickness care, maternal care, child care	Middle-level management skills Advanced medical skills and some public-health knowledge	MD with middle-level management training (certificate)
Surveillance program supervisor	Supervision of surveillance programs	Middle-level management skills Middle-level public-health skills	Senior nurse with middle-level management training (certificate)
Safe-water program supervisor	Supervision of safe-water program	Middle-level management skills Training in water safety	Environmental engineer with middle-level management training (certificate)
Safe-latrine and waste-disposal program supervisor	Supervision of safe-latrine and waste-disposal program	Middle-level management skills Training in latrine and waste-disposal problems	Environmental engineer with middle-level management training (certificate)
Health-education program supervisor	Supervision of health-education program	Middle-level management skills Training in health education	Health education (MPH) with middle-level management training (certificate)

flaws. First of all, the BHC is the most peripheral unit of large governmental ministries. BHCs are distributed widely in remote and difficult living environments. The abilities of developing countries to manage these remote, decentralized units is extremely limited. Poor roads, lack of telephone communications, and a poorly understood definition of operating procedures for BHCs contribute to ineffective management.

Second, the expected jobs of the BHC are too complex. The BHC is not a simple unit in most developing countries. It is first and foremost a medical unit for the care of sick people. This is its primary job, because this is what the people want and expect. They want relief from fear, pain, and suffering when sick. In addition, in most developing countries, the BHC is supposed to be the public-health department for its surrounding area. This function is almost never effective. Why is this?

One reason is that public-health programs are planned activities that require a degree of management sophistication not commonly found in the personnel assigned to the BHC. Second, inadequate numbers of personnel are assigned to do the public-health tasks at a minimum level of effectiveness. For a community of 25,000 people in the United States, there would be about 150 people involved in sickness care and over 100 involved in community public health, including water and sewer department personnel. How the BHC in Afghanistan is expected to make improvements in community health for 25,000 people with three medical workers and three public health workers is difficult to imagine.

Third, the training of workers is inadequate and inappropriate to their jobs at the BHCs. The doctor in particular is inappropriately trained. A job analysis of the doctor's job, as presently conceived, shows that up to 50 percent of his time should be spent in management-related activities. Yet doctors receive no management training and their technical training is urban-based and hospital-specific. How they can be expected to be effective BHC managers is also difficult to imagine.

The issues of BHC management need to be faced. Should a doctor with 7 years of technical training spend half his time in activities outside his field of training? Is he motivated? Is this the best use of his time? If the BHC is to fulfill community-health functions, perhaps a BHC manager should be trained to relieve the doctor of the administrative tasks of the BHC. The doctor and the administrator should jointly plan community programs, and the administrator should be responsible for their implementation. This administrator should have a college degree and specialized training in BHC management. However, as shown in subsequent paragraphs, the BHC needs to be redefined.

Fourth, the management of a Basic Health Center System, as presently conceived, is too complex a management task for most developing-country ministries. A well-developed BHC would have four or more medical-care programs and up to nine community-health programs. Each medical-care program and each community-health program have multiple subcomponents that require management control. The amount of information needed to manage this number of functions correctly is extremely large. The conversion of these data into processed information in a form for management decision making requires the analysis capabilities of the Basic Health Services Department to be at least moderately sophisticated. This situation is not likely to be found in personnel working in health ministries. In fact, the design of such an information system is a complex task that might take 3 years of high-level technical assistance to develop and field test before any management at all might occur.

In addition, the abilities of developing-country health ministries to respond to performance deficiencies are limited. Most of the required management-support systems to correct deficiencies are underdeveloped. These systems must be designed, field tested, and staff trained in such a way that all the systems begin to function well about the same time. This systems-analysis and design capability is usually missing, and the need for it is poorly perceived in health ministries dominated by doctors trained in hospital medicine.

Fifth, the financial constraints on poor countries limit the number of activities they can successfully pursue. Afghanistan was spending 40 cents per capita on health. Only 12 cents went to basic health services. To achieve anything with 12 cents per capita takes careful planning and cost-benefit types of analyses. These analyses are rarely done, so ambitious programs are underfinanced and hence understaffed. As a result, each program functions at less than minimum standards for possible effectiveness. Thus morale plummets, cynicism sets in, personnel begin to look out for themselves, and the system becomes corrupted.

What Should Be Done?

The goal of the health system is to provide sick people with relief from fear, pain, and suffering and to improve the health status of the people. For this to be done, people must receive medical services upon demand in the closest possible areas to their homes. The majority of sickness problems are simple ones and, as this project has shown, can be successfully handled by trained villagers. The job of the BHC is to be the first referral point for problems villagers themselves cannot solve. To do this job, the medical capabilities of the staff must be well developed through specific training for providing medical services in a BHC setting. They must have adequate supplies of emergency drugs at all times as well as well-functioning emergency equipment. BHC workers must have emergency and minor-surgical skills to be effective. The medical job should be the main job of a *streamlined and simplified BHC*. The job of the government is to develop as many of these low-cost units as possible and distribute them widely among the population to support trained villagers giving primary care.

The community public-health jobs are complex and require adequate manpower, skilled planners, and operations managers backed up by adequate management units with supervisory and evaluation capacity. In most developing-country settings, the health of the people would be better served by separating the public-health jobs from the BHC. In developed countries, with all the skills in higher levels, the public-health departments are kept separate from the medical units. It is unlikely that developing countries with lesser-trained personnel can do what developed countries cannot. The BHC should not have public-health jobs in the community. Other units should be developed that can refer community-health problems requiring sickness care to the BHC, but which can take care of other community-health problems themselves. In the financially deficient developing-country situation, each community-health activity should be carefully studied for manageability and cost-benefit, and only one or two activities should be implemented in the beginning. If this occurs, the managers will be able to grow in skills at the same rate the jobs require, and the personnel for each program will be sufficient to achieve minimum effectiveness.

Recommendations for BHCs and Public Health in Rural Developing Countries

The following recommendations are certainly applicable for the least-developed countries. Countries moderately to well-developed should consider adding other jobs to the BHC only if their management systems are adequately staffed and developed.

1. Simplify the BHC. Limit the number of services that the BHC performs to medical care at the BHC. Planned activities requiring community involvement should be limited to deliveries on request and tuberculosis defaulter follow-up.
2. Determine the numbers of personnel needed by an analysis of demand. The types of personnel should be doctor(s) if enough exist in the country or middle-level paramedical workers plus female health workers and perhaps another person such as a male nurse to assist with dressings and to do the tuberculosis follow-up.
3. Determine the standard drug lists for this unit and ensure adequate supplies and a resupply capacity. Determine the cost of this system to be effective, the manpower needs and skills, and the transport requirements and develop an effective system. Do not scrimp on this system. Budget it fully, and do it right.
4. Develop a standard medical equipment list for this simplified unit with equipment for emergency care and minor surgery. The BHC cannot just be a pill-dispensing operation.
5. Design and field-test management-control systems to monitor the qual-

ity of medical care rendered by the BHC. Medical-care standards must be developed, and performance must be compared with the standards. The analysis capability of the management units must be developed so that the data can be converted into tabular and graphical displays of processed information that compare performance with standards and trends over time. The complexity of this simplified information system will tax the capability of most developing-country ministries.

6. Make sure the ministry can take corrective actions for deficiencies found. Ensure that adequate positive and negative incentives exist to reward good work and punish poor work caused by lack of motivation. Have an adequate training capacity to remedy poor performance caused by lack of skills.

7. The training capacity of the management units for BHCs must be planned to be able to react to deficiencies found, but also to have standardized practical training to prevent skill decay and to give new skills. New skill development is not the primary function of a continuing-education unit. Basic skills must be developed in the basic training programs: medicine, nursing, and paramedical schools. Make sure that the budgets and manpower needs are met.

8. Conduct a careful cost-benefit analysis for community public-health programs. Determine the minimum budgets, manpower requirements (services and management-control personnel), transport requirements, and supply requirements for each program. Make a priority list of programs based on expected benefit, costs, and complexity of management. Determine, based on the budgets available, *how many* of these programs should be developed correctly. Do those and do not do the others until more budgets become available. An ineffective program is not worth doing.

9. Have an entirely separate services and management structure for the community public-health programs. Do not have the same managers attempt to manage the BHC and the community public-health programs. The nature of the jobs is very different.

10. Train public-health workers in management techniques as well as the content of public-health practice. Stress applied learning in the field. Carefully analyze overseas training programs to try to get programs with a primary management focus that use public-health knowledge to do things.

11. The final result will be numerous simplified BHCs spread throughout the country. They will provide medical backup to trained villagers who give the primary care in the villages. In addition, perhaps at different levels of population, there will exist public-health departments, separately managed, that will carry out one or more public-health programs based on the priority list and budget available. The public-health

departments will be managed best by a nonphysician college graduate with special training in public-health management.

Recommendations for Donor Planning and Phasing of
Projects in Rural Health

The following recommendations for donor planning and project phasing in rural health should increase both the effectiveness and efficiency of rural-health projects.

1. Consider carefully the recommendations made for the nature of the BHC and for management of the BHC.
2. Consider carefully the recommendations made for analysis and development of public-health programs, particularly the needs for each program to be adequately budgeted and staffed to perform at some predetermined minimum standard.
3. Think of projects in phases. Phase 1 should take from 1 to 2 years, and the following activities should occur:
    a. Send as many developing-country managers or potential managers abroad for basic management training related to medical care and public health in developing countries. These courses will be 1 to 2 years long.
    b. Send as many developing-country trainers or potential trainers abroad for training in technical areas of training: job analysis, training-objectives development, development of learning activities, course sequencing and planning, pedagogy (how to teach), and student evaluation and testing. These programs will take 1 to 2 years to complete.
    c. While workers are abroad receiving management and educational science training, have technical experts assist the government with a thorough analysis of the BHC's jobs, its personnel requirements, its management requirements, and its evaluation requirements. Develop predetermined minimum standards for all necessary management-influenced activities.
    d. Study the curricula of the basic training institutions for appropriateness to the needs of the country, and recommend changes.
    e. Conduct a thorough cost-benefit analysis, using technical experts, that will try to determine expected benefits in reducing mortality, morbidity, and disability by means of different public-health programs. Determine the budget and staffing requirements for each program to attain an acceptable minimum standard of effectiveness. Rank the programs and determine which should be attempted first.

Design carefully the service packages and management requirements for the planned programs, and, if possible, pick leaders and begin staff development training.

4. Phase 2 activities are implementation-related. By this time, the overseas trainees should have returned. They should not be involved in time-consuming educational advancement during implementation. If further people are to go abroad, they should be people who will be involved in phase 3 activities. Phase 2 will take 3 to 5 years, and the following activities will be undertaken:

   a. Involve the managers in the development of the medical-care management-control systems and develop, based on a priority list, the first management-control systems and plan for staff training and system start-up.

   b. Assist the basic training institutions in changing their programs to fit the needs of the country.

   c. Set up the continuing-education training unit and develop curricula based on a survey of deficiencies in skills of BHC workers. Do not develop curricula for problems caused by poor motivation and management. Begin training.

   d. Do the detailed design for the public-health programs that will be implemented. Consider the services requirements, the management requirements, and the staff-development requirements. Begin training of public-health department managers who are college graduates if possible. Their training in public-health management will take 9 months to a year. Begin implementation of top-priority program in the second year of phase 2. Do not add new services to public-health departments without careful analysis of the management-control requirements for any new service.

5. Phase 3 activities include the further improvement of the medical-care management-control systems and, if budget is available, the design and implementation of second-priority public-health programs. In addition, an evaluation of progress so far should occur with particular emphasis on improvements in the curricula of the basic training institutions and how their graduates, if any, are performing in the BHCs or the public-health department activities.

These recommendations should achieve an orderly development of the rural-health systems. Another requirement for the success of planned programs is political stability, but well-designed and implemented public-health systems should survive changes of governments.

Appendix E:
Training Methods of the National Traditional Midwife (*Dai*) Program of Afghanistan

John W. LeSar

One of the reasons that the National *Dai* Training Program in Afghanistan has been successful has been that an illiterate village *dai,* after the *dai* basic training course, can demonstrate to health professionals that she can take a medical history on a woman or child, perform a satisfactory physical examination for important physical signs, make a correct assessment of the severity of the problem, advise appropriate treatment (including referral), and give health education. How can an illiterate woman demonstrate these things after only 5 weeks of training? The answer lies in the *dai* training methods.

The National *Dai* Training Program uses a carefully organized approach to training based on an analysis of the jobs the *dai* must do in her environment. This organized approach has been called *training by objectives* or *criterion-referenced instruction* by educational experts. Besides being a carefully designed approach to training, this method of training gives detailed and specific information about how the program is doing—its weak points and its strong points. Thus the training managers can be responsible for many training teams and know how students in each program are doing for any given subject area of the curriculum (for example, prenatal care) or for any given process area of the curriculum (for example, history taking). This feedback information about student progress and performance allows immediate modifications to improve weak training areas, and the training programs steadily improve. In addition, because the curriculum is carefully designed and easily evaluated, it is easy for trainers to use. It is easy to *teach* the trainers how to use the curriculum, and it is easy to *evaluate* the trainers as well as the students.

The training methods will be described by their critical components, which are listed below. It is necessary that all these components be successfully addressed if high-quality, relevant training is to be achieved.

Job analysis

Development of training objectives

Course planning

Development of learning activities

Development of teaching materials

Development of student-evaluation methods

Teacher training

Good recruitment and selection methods

Good training environment

Support of the graduate

Feedback system for improvements

How the National *Dai* Training Program used this systematic approach in the training of village traditional midwives will be described in this section.

A. Job Analysis

Job analysis is the process of determining very specifically what the worker must do in a job. It compares the desired performance to the actual performance and, where discrepancies exist, develops task-mastery lists that guide the training process.

The program strategy, based on analyses of the health situation, the demographic situation, and the current and projected status of the government health system, led to the determination of the role and responsibilities of the *dai* in the overall plan for improving the health of the rural people of Afghanistan. The role of the *dai* is to provide primary health care to women and children under the age of 5 years in rural areas where access to the Basic Health Centers is difficult or where trained female health workers do not exist. The responsibilities, therefore, are to distinguish normal and not seriously sick people from high-risk and seriously sick people, to refer high-risk and seriously sick people to the Basic Health Center or hospital, and to offer treatment and health education to normal and not seriously sick people. From this definition of the role and responsibilities of the *dai* in the overall health system of Afghanistan, a list of desired performance skills was developed; the list follows.

Maternity Care

1. Prenatal care: Recognition of a normal from an abnormal or high-risk pregnancy; referral of the abnormal or high-risk pregnancy; nutritional

treatment of a normal pregnancy; health and nutritional education for the normal pregnancy.

2. Labor and delivery: Recognition of the normal from the abnormal labor; techniques of safe delivery of the vertex (head) presentation; techniques for safe delivery of the placenta; recognition of problems of the newly born baby; techniques of care of the newly born baby; referral of women with abnormal labor and/or delivery; referral of newly born babies with problems.

3. Postpartum care for mothers: Recognition of the postpartum woman with complications; referral of the postpartum woman with complications; education of the postpartum woman about breast care, nutrition while lactating, and hygiene.

4. Postpartum care for children up to 1 month of age: Recognition of the normal infant from the sick infant; referral of the sick infant; education of the mother about care of the infant in the first month of life.

5. Family-planning education: Reasons for family planning; methods of family planning; education of the mother about family planning.

Child Care for the Under-5 Child

1. Recognition of the normal, seriously sick, and not seriously sick child.
2. Tentative diagnoses for seventeen common conditions of childhood, including malnutrition:

Not Seriously Sick	*Seriously Sick*
Malnutrition without infection	Fever without other findings
Eye infection	Fever with malnutrition
Mild sore throat	Fever with rash
Mild cough	Fever with swelling
Mild diarrhea without dehydration	Fever with a full soft spot or stiff neck
Nondangerous skin infections	Fever with earache
Worms	Fever with pus in the throat
	Fever with difficult, rapid, wet breathing or cough with sputum
	Fever with painful or hard abdomen
	Dehydration

3. Treatment for five common conditions using nonprescription drugs and nutritional therapy; referral of other conditions.
4. Education of mothers of children about general care of the under-5

child; nutrition and feeding; prevention, recognition, and treatment of the child with diarrhea (including the preparation and use of oral rehydration materials); and prevention, recognition, and treatment of eye problems, skin problems, and worms.

From studies concerning the *dai* in rural Afghanistan, the following facts were known:

The average *dai* was about 50 years old

The clientele of the *dai* were generally from the same neighborhood

Dais learned skills from other *dais* (usually family members) and from observing and assisting many deliveries

Dais had some correct practices, helpful or harmful, and many poor practices, especially related to the mechanics of delivery

Thus, while the *dai* had much knowledge and experience, her skills were based on indigenous systems and were of uneven quality. There were also many gaps in her knowledge, attitudes, and practices. For this reason, the preceding list was adopted as the "task-mastery list" from which the basic curriculum would be derived.

After three or four training classes had been conducted, it was decided to add some other tasks to the task-mastery list of the basic course. These tasks were to develop interpersonal and health-education skills and are as follows:

Why people do things in certain ways

Why change takes a long time

How to find out problems

How to introduce new ideas

Thus the job analysis, based on the roles and responsibilities of the *dai* in the overall health system of Afghanistan, the actual performance of the *dai* in the rural areas at the time the program began, and early experiences in training of *dais* led to the task-mastery list from which the curriculum was derived.

B. Development of Training Objectives

The development of clear, concise behavioral objectives that specify the actions workers must do in their work, the conditions under which the actions are to be accomplished, and the minimum standard competencies for each task form the basis of the CRI approach to training. The training objectives are the roadmap that guides the teacher and student through the training process so that skills on the task-mastery list are transferred to the student at predetermined levels of quality.

The development of the training objectives is a difficult task for the training-program designer. If the training objectives are clear and concise, if each training objective builds on the successful mastery of the previous ones, and if gaps in fact or logic are avoided, the student can smoothly progress through the training course. If the objectives are not clear, carefully sequenced, and factually and logically consistent, the student becomes confused. This is why good design is critical to successful training.

If the training objectives satisfy the preceding conditions, the evaluation of student progress is easy because it derives directly from the training objectives and teaching points. The curriculum of the National *Dai* Training Program used this approach to provide the high-quality instruction necessary to train people with little or no formal education who work independently of better-trained health workers. How the *dai* curriculum was derived will be demonstrated in the following sections of this appendix.

An Example

If the reader looks again at the task-mastery list, the first task to be mastered is recognition of the normal from an abnormal or high-risk pregnancy. The job of the curriculum designer is to develop training objectives that, once mastered, will fulfill this task.

The National *Dai* Training Program curriculum divides this task of *problem recognition* into three topical areas. These are history taking, physical examination, and diagnosis. Through the use of the data-collection techniques of history taking and physical examination and using specified criteria for the diagnosis, the *dai* arrives at the correct answer. Thus, for the example of recognition of the normal from the abnormal or high-risk pregnancy, three training objectives were developed that describe the behaviors necessary to accomplish this task. These are shown in table E–1.

In other words, by asking specified questions and examining the pregnant woman for specified abnormal signs, the *dai* can collect the critical information. Once the information is collected, the *dai,* using the eleven criteria for recognition of the high-risk or abnormal pregnancy, makes the diagnosis of normal pregnancy, abnormal pregnancy, or high-risk pregnancy.

For each objective, there are a series of *teaching points*. The teaching points for the first two training objectives in prenatal care are shown in table E–2. The teaching points tell the *dai* exactly what to do. They are

Table E-1
Training Objectives for Recognition of the Normal from an Abnormal or High-Risk Pregnancy

Topic	Training Objective
History taking	1. Recite the seven questions to ask every pregnant woman
Physical Examination	2. Demonstrate the five abnormal signs to look for in every pregnant woman
Diagnosis	3. Recite the eleven points about how to recognize a high-risk or abnormal pregnancy

Table E-2
Teaching Points for the First Two Training Objectives in Prenatal Care

Topic	Training Objective
History-taking	Recite the seven questions to ask every pregnant woman
	Teaching Points
	1. How old are you?
	2. How many pregnancies have you had?
	3. Have you had bleeding?
	4. Have you had difficult deliveries?
	5. Are the rings on your hands too tight?
	6. Are you having frequent, bad headaches?
	7. Have you had a cough for more than 2 weeks or a cough with blood?
Physical Examination	Demonstrate the five abnormal signs to look for in every pregnant woman
	Teaching Points
	1. Observe the eyes, gums, and fingernails for paleness.
	2. Feel the abdomen to determine if the baby is sideways in the womb.
	3. Squeeze the hips together to determine if there is pain.
	4. Observe the face and hands for swelling.
	5. Measure the height by using reference mark to determine if the height is under 145 cm.

Table E–3
Teaching Points for the Third Training Objective in Prenatal Care

Topic	Training Objective
Diagnosis	Recite the eleven points about how to recognize an abnormal or high-risk pregnancy
	Teaching Points
	1. Age over 40 or under 16
	2. More than five pregnancies
	3. Bleeding from vagina
	4. History of difficult deliveries
	5. Swelling of hands so rings are tight
	6. Frequent severe headaches
	7. Very pale eyes
	8. Baby sideways in the womb
	9. Painful hips
	10. Shorter height than 145 cm
	11. Cough for more than 2 weeks

derived from the state of medical knowledge about normal, abnormal, and high-risk conditions and the epidemiologic situation of rural Afghanistan.

Once the *dai* knows the history questions and can do the physical exam, the third training objective gives the criteria for abnormal or high-risk women. The teaching points are shown in table E–3.

The reader can see the clarity, conciseness, careful sequencing, and factual and logical consistency of the training objectives. It is not difficult for the *dai* to make the diagnosis of normal, abnormal, or high-risk pregnancy once trained in this manner. Not only that, the training objectives are focused on the sequence of events the *dai* must perform to make the diagnosis, that is, ask questions and examine patients.

This approach works because of the epidemiology of maternal health problems. It is known that more than 80 percent of women will have normal pregnancies. The abnormal and high-risk groups contribute almost all the deaths and complications owing to pregnancy. Thus, using this approach, the *dai* can care for over 80 percent of cases and refer the abnormal or high-risk group to better-trained workers in, hopefully, better-equipped facilities.

Once the *dai* has made the diagnosis, she has two main categories of tasks to perform: give treatment (including referral) and give health education. For the abnormal or high-risk woman, the treatment is referral. For the normal pregnancy, the prenatal treatment is health education. Most of the remaining time is spent in health education. The remaining training objectives for prenatal care are shown in table E–4.

Thus the training objectives for the *dai* curriculum are divided into five topical areas: history taking, physical examinations, diagnosis, treatment, and health education. Each subject area of the curriculum uses this topical categorization. This repeating format makes learning easy for the *dai* because it is based on the sequence of events she must use with each patient. It is also critically important for evaluation, as will be shown later.

C. Course Planning

Once the training objectives are determined, the course designer must plan the organization of the course. This includes the development and sequencing of teaching units and the development of learning activities, as well as certain other considerations.

Development and Sequencing of Teaching Units

The *dai* training objectives fell into natural training units based on the job analysis and natural sequences of pregnancy and child care. The units were as follows:

Pregnancy care

    Prenatal care
    Labor and delivery
    Postpartum care for mothers
    Postpartum care for babies

Family-planning education

How to give health education

Medical care for the under-5 child

    Nutrition/malnutrition
    Diarrhea
    Eye problems
    Skin problems
    Throat and respiratory problems
    Worms
    Wound care
    Other selected problems

Table E-4
The Remaining Training Objectives for Prenatal Care

Topic	Training Objectives
Treatment	4. Recite one point about treatment of the abnormal or high-risk woman.
Education	5. Recite six teaching points about self-care during pregnancy
	6. Recite four teaching points about what the pregnant woman should eat every day
	7. Recite five points to tell the mother about danger signs of pregnancy
	8. Recite five teaching points about protection of the pregnant woman and her family from tuberculosis
	9. Recite five items to tell the mother to prepare for delivery

Other Considerations in Course Planning

There were certain considerations in the course planning process. These were as follows:

Training units should start with familiar areas and go to nonfamiliar areas.

The training units should be based on the learning process.

The training should be related to prevailing expectations.

The training should help build the training group.

The training should incorporate unifying themes.

The training units should be consistent.

Familiar to Nonfamiliar: With persons who are not used to formal training, it is important to begin with familiar topics. Thus the training program began with pregnancy care.

Based on Learning Process: The training units followed the natural course of pregnancy over time. Within each training unit, the natural process of investigating the problems of sick people was followed (history taking, physical exam, and so forth). Learning theory was followed by beginning with tasks involving simple recall (history taking), followed by more complex psychomotor tasks (physical exam), and then followed by the highest form of learning, synthesis (diagnosis). These natural sequences maximize the learning process.

Based on Prevailing Expectations: The training units did what the *dais* thought they would do—trained them in how to do their work in better ways. Theory was not prominent, nor was there unnecessary anatomic and physiologic detail.

Building the Training Group: It is important to build cohesiveness within the student group and between the teachers and the student group. This was accomplished by having the *dais* live together (some *dais* lived nearby to the course and did not stay overnight, but ate lunch at the class site), and with the teachers, by having *dai* training teams capable of teaching in two different languages, and by having an emphasis on group work during the training sessions.

Incorporating Unifying Themes: The unifying themes of the *dai* training course were the importance of health education, the importance of referral of serious or high-risk cases, and the importance of service to the community.

Consistency of Training Units: Considerable effort and many revisions were required to make each part of the *dai* curriculum internally consistent with and mutually reinforcing of every other part. This technical work is critically important in guaranteeing clear understanding of course material—particularly for health education—so that each *dai* gives similar messages on the subject matter.

Development of Learning Experiences

Learning experiences are situations in which the student will either experience the future work task under supervision or, in cases where direct experiences are difficult, will experience the task through simulation. The learning experiences are developed after the training objectives, and each set of learning is based on a training objective. The characteristics of good learning experiences are listed below:

They involve the student in the learning process; that is, the student actively participates in the learning task.

They break tasks into small steps and let students experience each step at a rate where successes are maximized.

They use practical, everyday examples to clarify teaching points.

They draw on students' backgrounds and own experiences to relate to subject matter.

They give students a chance to ask questions during experience.

They give students a chance to follow experience with reflection and discussions.

They repeat tasks with increasing responsibilities.

They use simulations effectively and maximize active participation.

They encourage value formation as well as skill development.

Examples of how the *Dai* Program followed these principles follow.

They Involve Students in the Learning Process: The teaching methods determine the extent of student involvement. Figure E–1 shows the differences in teaching methods from the passive-trainee role to the active-trainee role. From this figure it can be seen that lectures are the worst form of instruction and that direct supervised experience is the best. The examples from the *dai* curriculum shown in table E–5 illustrate the principles of active learning. In the *dai* curriculum, learning experiences in the teacher's guide are called "How to Teach This."

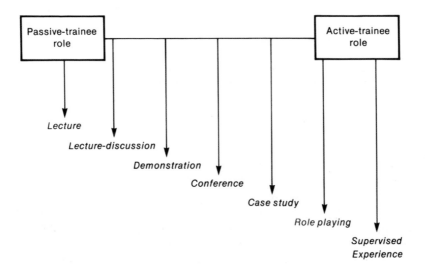

Figure E–1. Teaching Methods and Trainee Participation

Table E–5
Active Learning in the *Dai* Curriculum

Topic	Objectives and Teaching Points	How to Teach This
1.0 History taking	1.1 Recite the seven questions to ask every pregnant woman. *Teaching Points* 1. How old are you? 2. How many pregnancies have you had? 3. Have you had bleeding? 4. Have you had hard deliveries? 5. Are your rings too tight? 6. Are you having frequent bad headaches? 7. Have you had a cough for more than 2 weeks or a cough with blood?	1. Discuss why it is important to know about high-risk conditions. 2. Have the *dais* practice asking the seven questions of each other. 3. Have the *dais* practice asking the questions of pregnant mothers. 4. Have the *dais* memorize the seven history questions
2.0 Physical examination	2.1 To examine pregnant woman for five abnormal signs. *Teaching Points* 1. Observe eyes, gums, and skin for paleness. 2. Feel abdomen to determine if baby is sideways in womb. 3. Squeeze hips together to determine if there is pain. 4. Observe face and hands for swelling. 5. Measure height by using reference mark on *dai* (145 cm) to determine if height is under 145 cm.	1. Discuss the five physical signs of high-risk and the *dai*'s experience. 2. Have *dais* perform exams on each other and on instructors. 3. Perform examination on pregnant patients, including height of patient.

It can be seen that discussions and supervised practice are the predominant learning modes. Role playing was often used to act out the learning experience. This was a favorite learning experience of the *dais,* who loved to pretend they were in the village. One *dai* would often be the patient, and another the *dai,* as they demonstrated how they handled problems. *Dais* actually used clothes and even turbans to make role playing more realistic. *Dais* did not mind pretending to be men. Table E–6 illustrates the use of stories and case studies.

It is also important to have repetition of critical steps in the learning process. Overlearning and constant repetition under supervision are impor-

Table E-6
The Use of Stories and Case Studies in the *Dai* Curriculum

Topic	Objectives and Teaching Points	How to Teach This
3.0 Diagnosis	3.1 Recite eleven points about how to recognize a high-risk pregnancy. *Teaching Points* 1. Age over 40 or under 16 2. More than five pregnancies 3. Bleeding from vagina 4. Difficult deliveries 5. Swelling of hands so rings are tight 6. Frequent severe headaches 7. Very pale eyes 8. Baby sideways in womb 9. Painful hips 10. Shorter height than mark on *dai* 11. Cough over 2 weeks or cough with blood	1. Tell stories or case studies about pregnant women and have *dais* decide whether pregnancy is normal or high-risk 2. Have *dais* diagnose high-risk pregnancy by asking history questions and by examinations. 3. Have *dais* tell stories of their experiences.
4.0 Treatment	4.1 Recite one point about treatment of the high-risk pregnant woman. *Teaching Point* 1. Refer high-risk women to the health center or hospital	1. Discuss patients and create stories of pregnant women who are high-risk or normal. 2. Discuss traditional treatments and discourage harmful ones.

tant in the training of people with little or no prior education. The preceding tables demonstrate the use of repetition of previous steps.

They Break Tasks into Small Steps: The progression of teaching objectives and learning experiences is sequential, with each task building on the previous skill. In the preceding tables, the progression from history taking to physical examination to diagnosis to treatment is shown. Table E-7 finishes this particular sequence.

They Use Practical, Everyday Examples to Clarify Teaching Points: The use of role playing and story telling allows the teachers to let the *dais* learn using their own experiences. The learning experiences from the diagnosis and treatment sections demonstrate this point.

They Draw on Students' Backgrounds and Own Experiences: The use of role playing and story telling also demonstrate the use of the student's own experiences.

Table E–7
The Final Sequence of Teaching Points in the *Dai* Curriculum for
Pregnancy and Child Care

Topic	Objectives and Teaching Points	How to Teach This
5.0 Education	5.1 Recite five teaching points about self-care during pregnancy.	1. Ask *dais* what they do.
		2. Encourage good points.
	Teaching Points	3. Teach five points about self-care.
	1. Do not wear tight clothes.	4. Have *dais* practice on each other (role playing).
	2. Bathe at least two times a week.	
	3. Rest frequently by lying down with feet up.	5. Have *dais* practice on patients.
	4. Smoke less.	6. Demonstrate vaseline application.
	5. From 7 months of pregnancy, massage breasts with vaseline each night and wash breasts each morning (mainly primapara).	7. Practice recitation for memorization.
	5.2 Recite four teaching points about protection of mother and family from tuberculosis.	1. Ask the *dais* what they do in their practice.
		2. Encourage good practices.
	Teaching Points	3. Teach the four points about protection.
	1. Cover mouth when coughing because tuberculosis is spread through the air.	4. Have *dais* practice on each other (role playing).
	2. Clean clothes of a tuberculosis pattient separately from the rest of the family.	5. Have *dais* practice on patients.
		6. Practice reciting the teaching points for memorization.
	3. Do not cough in baby's face when breastfeeding.	7. Explain that tuberculosis is transmitted by air most of the time.
	4. A person with active tuberculosis must sleep and eat apart from the family. The person should not kiss babies or children.	
	5.3 Recite four teaching points about what the pregnant women should eat every day.	1. Discuss why foods are important: body building, energy, protection.
		2. Discuss costs for their patients and what women eat and why.
	Teaching Points	3. Have *dais* shop for food and fix a balanced diet meal.
	1. Eat yoghurt or drink milk.	
	2. Eat vegetables and fruits.	4. Emphasize importance of gaining weight.
	3. Eat meat, liver, eggs, or WFP rations.	5. Demonstrate use of WFP rations.
	4. Eat bread or cereal.	

Table E-7 (continued)

5.4 Recite five items to tell the mother to prepare for delivery
 	
Teaching Points
1. Clean, sun-dried cloth and plastic cloth.
2. Small cloth for wrapping baby.
3. One new razor blade.
4. One large basin for bathing the baby.
5. Prepare thread and gauze.
	1. Demonstrate how to clean the cloth, dry cloth, cut cloth, and store it for each type of use:
	  a. for cord
	  b. for under mother at delivery
	  c. for baby
	  d. for baby's eyes
	  e. for perineal pads
	2. Demonstrate how to pack a cord kit:
	  a. razor blade
	  b. thin cloth for cord
	3. Practice for each *dai* at least two times.

They Give Student a Chance to Ask Questions during Experience: The discussion sessions are interactive; that is, the student and the teachers interact together. The discussions in the *Dai* Program encourage questions, and the use of another trained *dai* as a teacher reduces the shyness of students in asking questions.

They Give Students a Chance to Follow Experience with Reflection and Discussions: The training environment of the *Dai* Program was designed to use the evenings for reflection and discussions. The students and teachers lived together, ate together, and relaxed together in the evening, where talk often turned to problems of pregnancy and children, and where students considered their learning experiences and discussed their day with fellow students. It often seemed that as much learning occurred in the evening as during the day, and the evening sessions contributed greatly to value formation and feelings of positive self-worth.

They Repeat Tasks with Increasing Responsibility: Since the training is sequentially developed, the students practice each prior step while learning the new one. The students also begin practicing on themselves, then on plastic pelvic models or babies, as needed, and then on people at the BHC or local hospital. As training progresses, the experiences are repeated with less instructor supervision so that by graduation, independent assessment, treatment, and education are being done.

They Use Simulation Effectively and Maximize Active Participation: Certain training objectives cannot be met by supervised experience. Therefore,

Table E–8
The Use of Simulation in the *Dai* Curriculum

Topic	Objectives and Teaching Points	How to Teach This
4.0 Treatment	4.2 Tell and demonstrate the two things the *dai* should do during delivery.	1. Demonstrate with pelvic model. 2. Trip to hospital to observe delivery.
	Teaching Points 1. In head presentation, place one hand on baby's head to guide the birth and prevent tears. 2. Check for cord around the neck. 3. If loose, pull cord over head. If tight, complete delivery.	
	4.3 Tell and demonstrate the two things the *dai* should do immediately after delivery of the baby before cutting the cord.	1. Have each *dai* practice action in sequence model.
	Teaching Points 1. Turn baby upside down to allow fluids to drain out. 2. See if baby is breathing normally.	
	4.4 Tell and demonstrate the four steps the *dai* should use when cutting the cord before delivery of the placenta.	1. Practice with model.
	Teaching Points 1. Tie the cord one finger away from the baby. 2. Clamp the cord on the side closest to the mother. 3. Cut the cord between the tie and the clamp. 4. Cover with a clean cloth.	

simulations should be used to involve the student in active learning. Table E–8 illustrates the effective use of simulation in the *dai* curriculum.

They Encourage Value Formation: The use of story telling, case studies, and reflection and discussion contribute to value formation. By graduation, *dais* feel themselves to be an important health resource to their village.

Table E-9
Teaching Materials in the *Dai* Teacher's Guide

How to Teach This	Teaching Materials
1. Discuss why foods are important: body building, energy, protection	1. Examples of each kind of food, have a free lunch with a balanced meal for a pregnant woman. *Dais* should buy the food.
2. Discuss costs for their patients and what women eat and why	
3. Have *dais* shop for food and fix a balanced meal	1. WFP rations
	3. Cooking utensils
4. Emphasize importance of gaining weight	4. Money
5. Demonstrate use of WFP rations.	

1. Demonstrate how to clean the cloth, dry cloth, cut cloth, and store it for each type of use.
  a. for cord
  b. for under mother at delivery
  c. for baby
  d. for baby's eyes
  e. for perineal pads
	1. Soap from bazaar
	2. Basin
	3. Cloth
	4. Scissors from midwifery kit
	5. Razor blade

2. Demonstrate how to pack a cord kit:
  a. razor blade
  b. thin cloth for cord	

3. Practice for each *dai* at least two times	

D. Development of Teaching Materials

The development of teaching materials is important to illustrate points where supervised practical experiences are difficult. The instructor must plan ahead so that he or she has the required materials at the time of teaching. Table E-9 demonstrates how teaching materials are incorporated into the teacher's guide.

E. Development of Student-Evaluation Methods

The evaluation of health-worker training is important, particularly for village-based workers. There must be conclusive evidence that the worker has skills to implement acceptable quality primary care in the village. The *Dai* Program had a strong evaluation system—both in individual performance evaluation and in analysis of group-performance data to modify the teaching program. The following types of skill evaluation of *dais* were done: technical skills and interpersonal skills.

Technical Skills

The evaluation of technical skills involved evaluation of knowledge skills (recall, discrimination, synthesis) and manipulative skills (how to do things with one's hands). The *Dai* Program used both *test-measurement instruments* and *non-test-evaluation instruments* to evaluate technical skills.

The program used an oral pretest and posttest instrument to evaluate student progress in knowledge skills over the course of the program. The example is from the evaluation of prenatal care. It can be seen how this carefully follows the training objectives and teaching points as these stress practical application of knowledge needed to deal with patients. The evaluation was given orally, thus allowing both pretests and posttests to be on the same page.

The principle of criterion-referenced instruction is illustrated in the evaluation form in figure E–2. Each test question has criteria for passing. Thus each student receives a pass or fail on each question, and the number of questions answered correctly (criteria satisfied) becomes the score of the student. As will be demonstrated later, group analysis using this format gives extremely good information about the aggregated data, that is, the whole class. Therefore, the evaluation is useful for individual scoring and for group analysis.

The program also uses three non-test-measurement instruments, which are the anecdotal record, the checklist, and the rating scale. The *anecdotal record* is a factual report of a significant incident in a student's performance. For example:

> The *dai,* Gul Bibi, was observed by me at the Basic Health Center during her fifth week of training. She was examining a pregnant woman who came for a checkup. While talking with the woman, she found that the woman had been coughing for 3 months. The nurse said not to worry about it, but Gul Bibi was worried and called the doctor, who found tuberculosis. Gul Bibi's performance was excellent in both diagnosis and in being concerned enough about her patient to ask the doctor, even though the nurse said not to worry.
>
> Signed,
>
> Nurse Gulgotai
> Supervisor

The usefulness of the anecdotal record depends on the skill of the observer. Single anecdotes are seldom valuable, but anecdotes by many different observers are very valuable in assessing performance.

PRETEST DATE ___			QUESTIONS	POST TEST DATE ___			
Results (Pass / Fail)	Criteria For Passing	Check Box if Answer Is Correct		Check Box if Answer Is Correct	Criteria For Passing	Results (Pass / Fail)	

QUESTIONS

1. What 7 questions should you ask every pregnant woman?
   Answers:
   1. How old are you?
   2. How many pregnancies have you had?
   3. Have you had bleeding?
   4. Have you had hard deliveries?
   5. Are your rings too tight?
   6. Are you having frequent bad headaches?
   7. Have you had a cough for more than 2 weeks or a cough with blood?

   Criteria for Passing: 5 of 7 Answers Correct

2. When you examine a pregnant woman, what are 5 abnormal signs you should check for?
   Answers:
   1. Observe eyes, gums, and skin for paleness.
   2. Feel abdomen to determine if baby is sideways in womb.
   3. Squeeze hips together to determine if there is pain.
   4. Observe face and hands for swelling.
   5. Measure height by using reference mark on dai (145 cm) to determine if height is under 145 cm.

   Criteria for Passing: 4 of 5 Answers Correct

Figure E-2. *Dai* Evaluation: Prenatal Care 1

Form OBV-CC-1	DAI TRAINING-CHILD CARE SECTION OBSERVATION ON PATIENTS				
RECOGNITION OF ABNORMAL SIGNS			Dai Name Maria		
	FIRST WEEK		SECOND WEEK		
Abnormal Signs	Recognized	Not Recognized	Recognized	Not Recognized	Comments
Very Sick Child					
Fever					
Rash					
Swelling					
Full Soft Spot					
Stiff Neck					
Red Eyes					
Red Throat with Pus					

Figure E–3. *Dai* Training-Program Checklist

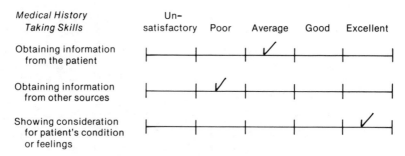

Figure E–4. *Dai* Training-Program Rating Scale

The *checklist* is a list of words, sentences, phrases, or paragraphs describing specific aspects of behavior to be evaluated during observation of a student at work. Figure E–3 is an example of a checklist.

The checklist must contain the critical skills to be evaluated. When constructing a checklist, think of the skills mentioned earlier: recall, discrimination, synthesis, manipulation, speech, and nonverbal communication.

The *rating scale* is a checklist with judgments added. Figure E–4 is such a rating scale. The advantages of the rating scale are that it gives more information than the checklist. The disadvantages are that judgments vary among observers. Four types of judges may be picked: experts (for example, teachers), peers (for example, students), clients (for example, people upon whom the service is performed), and self (for example, the student herself). Ratings tend to vary within judging groups and between judging groups, but the best use of rating scales involves judges of all four types.

Interpersonal Skills

The *Dai* Program has also used interpersonal evaluation, which is evaluation of communications skills (speech and nonverbal communication). The *dais* were sensitized to the importance of communications through health-education training with emphasis on communications processes. The *dais* actually discussed how people change their ideas and practiced communications methods on themselves and on patients. Table E–10 presents examples of interpersonal-evaluation indicators.

Interpersonal-skills evaluation is extremely important in knowing that the trained *dai* interacts with patients in such a way as to increase her effectiveness and her number of clients.

Group Evaluation

The *dai* curriculum and its testing methods were designed for easy group evaluation. Group evaluation is important for the following reasons:

Assessing strengths and weaknesses of particular classes

Assessing the performance of different training teams

Assessing the strengths and weaknesses in the curriculum that require modification

One group evaluation form is shown in figure E–5. It can be used to analyze both pretests and posttests as well as the basic course or continuing education (where all *dais* undergo thorough retesting to check their skills about 1 year after the basic course).

Of importance is that the curriculum can be evaluated by content areas or by process areas. This is illustrated below:

Pregnancy-Care Content-
Evaluation Areas

1. Prenatal Care (PNC)
2. Labor and delivery (L&D)
3. Postpartum care for the child (PPC)
4. Postpartum care for the mother (PPM)

Process-Evaluation Areas

1. History taking
2. Physical examination
3. Diagnosis
4. Treatment
5. Health education

Table E-10
Interpersonal-Evaluation Indicators

Effectiveness of Dai-Patient Relationship

A. Showing concern and consideration

Component-Skill Categories

1. Showing personal interest and concern
2. Acting in a discreet, tactful, and professional manner
3. Avoiding needless discomfort, alarm, or embarassment
4. Speaking honestly to patient and family

B. Relieving patient or family tensions

Component-Skill Categories

1. Reassuring or calming
2. Explaining condition, treatment, or prognosis

C. Improving patient cooperation

Component-skill categories

1. Persuading patient to undertake needed care
2. Insisting or remaining firm about needed care

Responsibility as a Trained Dai

A. Accepting Responsibility for Welfare of Patient

Component-skill categories

1. Heeding the call for help
2. Devoting necessary time and effort
3. Meeting commitments
4. Insisting on primacy of patient welfare
5. Delegating responsibility wisely

B. Recognizing professional capabilities and limitations

Component-skill categories

1. Doing only what experience permits
2. Asking for help, advice or consultation
3. Following instructions and advice
4. Showing conviction and decisiveness
5. Accepting responsibility for own error

C. Relating effectively to other health persons

Component-skill categories

1. Supporting the actions of other health workers
2. Maintaining open and honest communication
3. Helping other health workers
4. Relating in discreet, tactful manner
5. Respecting the physician's responsibility to his patient.

Average scores for this class evaluated during continuing education for both content analysis and process analysis are shown in figure E-5. It can be seen that the *dai*'s were weakest in family planning and in history taking before continuing education, but were above after continuing education. This information is compared with other classes. If the weak trends hold,

Basic Course

Continuing Education

Pregnancy Care/Health Education
Basic Training Curriculum: Pre-test/Post Test

% Students Passing Basic Training Post-Test

Dai Training Information System

TD#8   July 1978

Basic Course Evaluation Form (Pregnancy/Health Ed.)

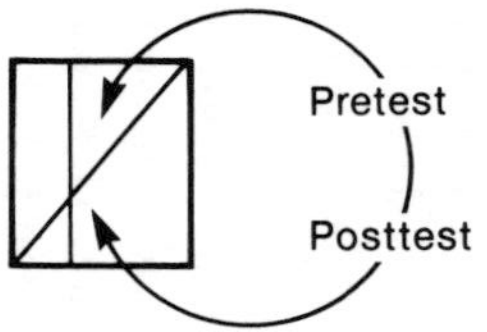

Pretest

Posttest

85 ———— Minimum Standard

Traditional Midwife Training Program
Presidency of Basic Health Services
Ministry of Public Health
Democratic Republic of Afghanistan

	ANC	L&D	PP-C	PP-M	F.P.	Average
History	76 / 100	86 / 100	67 / 100	90 / —	▒	80 / 98
Physical Examination	86 / 100	71 / 100	76 / 100	95 / —	▒	82 / 99
Diagnosis	100 / —	100 / —	100 / —	90 / —	▒	98 / 98
Treatment	100 / —	100 / —	100 / —	100 / —	▒	100 / 100
Health Education	100 / —	▒	76 / 100	100 / —	48 / 97	81 / 99
Average	92 / 100	89 / 100	84 / 100	95 / 95	48 / 97	99

Class   Balkh 1
Location   Balkh
Date of Training   July 1978
Evaluator   Reza

Comments on Pregnancy/Health Ed Section
This class had no manual or cassette or any other way to review. The basic course was 10 months ago. Considering no review mechanism, they did well.

Figure E-5. *Dai* Evaluation Program

the curriculum is analyzed in these areas, revised, and field-tested until improvements occur.

As a matter of interest, this particular continuing-education evaluation (along with the child-care evaluation not shown) pointed out the need for *dais* to have some reference material to study during the interim periods when they were in practice. Based on these data, a manual was developed that could be read by a literate member of the *dai*'s family so that she could refresh her memory.

As the *Dai* Program expands, supervision of the teachers will become a critical factor in the rate of expansion. Quality must be maintained if decentralized training is to exist on a large scale. This evaluation method allows program managers to compare training teams. For example, if Nazaneen's team over five classes has an average posttest score of 86 while Nasima's has 96, then the program-management staff should investigate why Nazaneen's performance is lower. Supervisory personnel can observe her team's teaching until scores improve.

Thus the curriculum and the evaluation systems are synergistically designed so that analysis is easy and modifications in the training or supervisory process can result in constant program improvement.

F. Teacher Training

Teacher training or staff development was discussed in chapter 3.

G. Good Recruitment and Selection Methods

Dai recruitment is based on securing approval of government representatives and village leaders before attempting to influence the *dai* herself. The *dai* recruitment team first visits the important officials (such as the provincial governor or the *woleswal*) in the small town where training usually takes place. If the local official agrees to participate in recruitment, he then sends out a message to the important village leaders in his region. After the village leaders have assembled (in the governor's or *woleswal*'s office), the *dai* recruitment team explains the program to them and answers their questions. The village leaders are then asked to return to their villages and help choose *dais* for the program. The exact starting date and place for the *dai* course are also explained to the leaders so that the *dais* will know where and when to go for the course. In addition, the *dai* recruitment teams visit those large villages located too far away from the training site for the village leaders to have attended the meeting. When the *dais* come to the training site to begin the course, each is interviewed by the *dai* recruitment team. If the woman has not had extensive experience delivering babies, if she is too old or senile, or if she is sick, she is rejected for the course.

The experience to date in recruiting over 540 *dais* can be summarized as follows. Despite great concern at the program's outset that Afghan village traditional birth attendants (*dais*) would be difficult to recruit, this has not turned out to be the case. Although Afghan village men are highly protective toward their women, recruitment targets thus far have always been met. There are several possible explanations for this. Most *dais* are older, so that village men may not be as concerned about protecting them as they would be about younger women, although, since the program has become well known, the age is dropping and women in their early thirties are common. Another explanation is that the village men are reassured that the women will be very safe living (in most cases) in a rented house surrounded by a protective wall, with every attention paid to their safety and comfort.

The most serious difficulties in recruiting *dais* have been political, particularly in 1979. Because of a long-standing and traditional mistrust that exists between rural and tribal Afghans, on the one hand, and the central Afghan government, on the other, many villagers are afraid that a government-sponsored program for training *dais* has some other, more sinister, purpose. This problem has not been insoluble, and repeated visits to a village by an obviously sincere recruitment team tends to soften local suspicions.

Perhaps the key factor in gaining village acceptance was gaining the trust and confidence of village men. Although Afghanistan has many ethnic groups, rural villagers share fairly common views about the role of women. The predominant view is that females should be secluded once they reach puberty and should not spend time with adult males outside of their family structure. This is expressed in varying degrees in different parts of the country, but the effect is that women usually remain within their housing compounds unless they are working with their husbands in the field, washing clothes, bringing water, or doing other domestic activities. In fact, it is often difficult for women to go to the Basic Health Center, even if accompanied by their husbands. The 5-week training course required many *dais* to leave their homes for the first time. Men were "won over" in the following ways:

Older women were recruited (30 to 60 years old) in early classes.

The *dais* were transported from their villages (or near their villages) to the training site, which was within the general region of their homes (mobile training sites).

The training site was in a walled compound, and men, other than the training staff, were not allowed in (including husbands who could come only to the door of the compound).

When the women left the compound, they were usually in a vehicle and remained in *chadri.*

Women left the compound only to go to the hospital, Basic Health Center, or family-guidance clinic.

The *dais* were trained separately from any male village workers.

After training, the *dais* were transported back to their village.

Another lesson learned during *dai* recruitment efforts was that local Afghan officials should not attempt recruiting of *dais.* Rather, a well-trained *dai* recruitment team (based in Kabul or at a regional training center) should have that responsibility. In one province where the Governor and other officials took responsibility for *dai* recruitment, many of the women selected turned out to have had no experience delivering babies and were found to be relatives of the officials doing the recruitment.

H. Good Training Environment

A good training environment is necessary to maximize learning. The *dai* basic training courses were extremely careful to develop and maintain a protective, supportive environment during the 5-week training courses.

Many *dais* had never lived away from their families. Many had never traveled even the relatively short distances to the training sites, which, using mobile training teams, were always located in rural BHCs or small towns that served a surrounding rural community. Most *dais* were in *chadri,* a piece of clothing that completely covered them when they were in public, including their faces and heads. They were extremely shy about public travel.

The *dai* trainers usually rented a house in the rural area or in a small town. The house had a surrounding wall, and the teachers and students lived together. The basic didactic training, using the active-learning techniques discussed earlier, took place in the rented house or outside the house, but inside the protective wall. The *dais* were thus relieved of having to study in public. The *dais* were never trained with male students, although male supervisors could visit without difficulty.

For patient-related training, the *dais* traveled by vehicle to the Basic Health Center or small hospital where the patients were. During maternal and child health days at the BHCs or small hospitals, there were usually a large number of women and children. In that public environment *dais* were comfortable because other women were present. Based on these methods, the *dais* were comfortable in their training environment.

One innovation of the program has been to also use trained *dais* as trainers. They are able to relate to fellow villagers and to bridge any communication gaps between the other *dai* trainers and the students. Their value as role models cannot be overemphasized, because they demonstrate the government's acceptance of well-trained *dais*. They also demonstrate that intelligent village women, even if illiterate, can make important contributions to their country.

Living together for 5 weeks encouraged an intense socialization process among the *dais* and trainers. These social bonds helped each *dai* be more comfortable with learning, particularly emotionally laden material such as discussions on sexual issues and family planning. This socialization process prevented the more urban nurse-midwife trainers from stressing the student role too much.

The training environment also fostered reflection and discussions, as mentioned earlier. While relaxing in the evenings, *dais* could discuss their experiences with other *dais*, reflect on their new skills, and interact with teachers, who shared cooking and cleanup duties. The importance of this group interaction was very important to the success of the program.

I. Support of the Graduate

The newly graduated *dai* must readjust to her home environment after her training. The drivers first took them to the Basic Health Center nearest their home to meet the doctor. The doctor had often participated in their recruitment, but it was important to know that he understood that a successful graduate had returned.

Within 1 year after training, the *dais* returned to a training site for 1 week of continuing education. The support program would have been improved by twice-yearly continuing education, but manpower and financial constraints prohibited this. During the continuing-education week, a detailed plan was followed.

Continuing-Education Week Activities

Day 1:   Give the posttest from the basic course; spend one-half day on discussions of problems faced by the *dais* in their work.

Day 2:   Review of entire basic course.

Day 3:   Indepth review of weak areas found by the posttest; interview each *dai* individually about her problems and successes.

Day 4:   New skills development using continuing-education modules

Day 5:   Final discussions about what it is like to be a *dai* working in the village.

The objectives of continuing-education week were threefold: first, to assess skill decay and reteach areas where it has occurred; second, to support the work and emotional life of the *dai* working in her village; and third, to conduct interviews about *dai* practices, utilization, and feelings about her work. Taped interviews have been done to assess the *dai*'s feelings about the following areas:

Taped Interviews to Assess Feelings

What happened to you when you returned to the village? (six questions)

How do people feel about you now? (eight questions)

What is the best way to introduce you to the village? (one question)

What are your biggest problems in your work? (one question)

What is the best part of your work in the village? (one question)

Are you happy with the amount of money you receive from your work? (one question)

What is your relationship with the BHC staff? (seven questions)

How could we improve the *dai* training program? (eight questions)

How do you feel about yourself? (five questions)

In this way, the program hopes to understand the *dai* and her problems in daily living and work. From these data, the training can be made more realistic and more supportive.

J. Feedback System for Improvements

The *dai* field-evaluation system is still in the research stage. Certain methods have been used, and other areas are in the design phase. Field evaluation is used to evaluate the practices of trained *dais* in their village and to assess the *dai* herself—her type of practice and her feelings toward her work. Development of the field-evaluation program was the primary developmental effort of the National *Dai* Program staff during 1979. It was hampered by lack of security in the rural areas.

Two instruments have been tested and used so far. One is the *dai* utilization survey. In this survey, assessments were made of the type of practice the *dais* had as well as how busy they were. Early data showed the following.

In a 2-week period, 87 percent of *dais* will see one or more sick children (95 percent of the time in the child's home); 67 percent of *dais* will see one or more pregnant women (87 percent of the time in the woman's home); 52 percent of *dais* will find at least one high-risk child that they refer to the BHC; 48 percent of *dais* will advise at least one woman about family planning; and 33 percent of *dais* will do at least one delivery.

In a 1-year period, *dais* do the following ("busy" *dais* are defined as being in the busiest third of the class):

	Busy Dai	*Average Dai*	
Visits related to pregnancy	203	125	
Visits related to child care	156	135	
Visits related to family planning	152	78	
Referrals of high-risk children to the BHC or hospital	52	20	(86 percent went)
Deliveries	31	17	
Referrals of high-risk mothers to the BHC or hospital	3.8	2.1 (74 percent went)	

In 1-year period, the activities of the **dais** are as follows:

	Busy Dai	*Average Dai*
Pregnancy-related activities	40%	37%
Child-care-related activities	30%	40%
Family-planning activities	30%	23%
Total	100%	100%

This preliminary information will be collected on larger samples of *dais*. Group profiles will be developed in a manner similar to the student-evaluation methods. In addition, consultant help is underway to evaluate the villagers' feelings about the *dais* and how *dais* practice in the field. Anthropologic and evaluation experts are assisting in this, and results should be available in about a year if the rural security situation improves. The objective of all field-evaluation activities is the ensure a happy, busy, trained *dai* doing high-quality work for her fellow villagers.

The National *Dai* Training Program of Afghanistan has used a systematic approach to training and evaluating its students that has produced a qualified primary worker of proven skills after 5 weeks of training. The careful development of the curriculum maximizes the amount of learning, so adult women with no prior schooling can progress rapidly in a series of small steps. The evaluation methods ensure skills and give information for improvement of the training process.

In the summer of 1978, a United Nations expert team did an evaluation of the program. The training specialist had these words to say: "In general, the program is sophisticated and well-structured, very complete in terms of technical/medical content. The training plan and other related materials are the most impressive the writer has ever seen."

The National *Dai* Training Program of Afghanistan has been an unqualified success in demonstrating that villagers can learn and have much to contribute. Afghan leaders have realized that the strength of the country is in its people, and the National *Dai* Training Program has contributed to this goal.

K. Summary

The development and stabilization of the National *Dai* Training Program has been dependent on the creation of a sound organization capable of securing and maintaining authority and resources. The development of program leadership, clear organizational objectives, sound technical training methods that are consistent with the needs of society, and a well-defined and functional organizational structure have contributed to the success of the program thus far.

After 2 years, the program is fairly stable. The MOPH constituency remains supportive, even though the government has changed. As of now, organizational leadership of the program is stable under the new government. Power battles over program control may continue, but the organizational structure of the program seems likely to remain intact. Other training organizations have not been sanctioned. The donor community remains pleased with the program and has supported expansion as requested by the government. Some donors are interested in having *Dai* Programs in other countries, based on experiences in Afghanistan. The village constituency, even with political turbulence, has continued to accept this program as a beneficial one.

Program stabilization has been greatly enhanced by international recognition. Visits to Afghanistan have been numerous by experts in health. Senior officials from WHO, UNDP, UNFPA, UNICEF, the World Bank, USAID, and other agencies have visited the *Dai* Program and have enthusiastically endorsed it. Two publications about Afghan *dais* have appeared in international journals, and the program was discussed at the WHO/UNICEF World Conference on Primary Health Care held at Alma Alta, U.S.S.R.

The National *Dai* Training Program has contributed toward the specified needs of society in these ways. First, it improves health in the village. Second, it upgrades an indigenous resource of the village. Third, it contributes toward a specialization of labor within the village, a necessary prerequisite to development. Fourth, it contributes toward changing the role and status of women, another necessary prerequisite for modernization. Fifth, it provides role models for young girls in the village.

The National *Dai* Training Program also has contributed to changing the image of the villager as a tradition-bound, unteachable person. Overall, the *dais* have been intelligent, eager to learn, and eager to adopt new ideas that make sense to them. Some *dais* have been trained as teachers and can now use modern teaching techniques to assist other *dais*. The National *Dai* Training Program has helped Afghan decision makers realize that the strength of their country lies in its citizens and that minimal investment costs give high benefits when applied to the rural people of Afghanistan.

Problems will always occur, but the National *Dai* Training Program seems likely to continue as an integral part of an improved rural health-care system for Afghanistan. So far, over 500,000 rural people have benefited, and millions more are likely to do so.

Appendix F:
Planning and Manpower
Development: Areas of
Frustration and Failure

The Ministry was aware that real constraints existed in their ability to plan and staff whatever programs were likely to emerge. As noted in figure 1–3, the initial workplan included efforts to improve the planning function and the personnel system, which was an essential initial step in manpower planning. Both activities were among the early failures of the project and continue to have a negative impact.

A. The Planning Department

The team was initially headquartered in the Planning Department, with members placed in other administrative and technical departments. The Planning Department encompassed three quite disparate entities: the Secretariat for the Planning Board, the Foreign Relations Office, and the Construction Directorate.

Although prominently placed on the Ministry organizational chart, the Planning Board had little creative force and acted primarily as a forum for its members, the senior officials from most Ministry departments and a few powerful institutions such as the Kabul hospitals. Board actions had little impact on Ministry direction, and large amounts of time were consumed on planning exercises often stimulated by government directives and donors, but without any linkage to Ministry operations. Foreign Relations was formally charged with responsibility for all interactions with donors, but generally played a ceremonial role once projects and individuals became acquanted with the Ministry. The Construction Directorate provided technical supervision of capital (development) projects.

Plans to alter this situation were enthusiastically developed in collaboration with Planning Department colleagues who saw the need and opportunity to upgrade their efforts. Despite initial Ministry approval to undertake the process, proposals to realign functions, upgrade staff, and introduce senior Ministry leadership failed to be enacted.

Two reasons for this failure seemed evident. First, senior Ministry officials correctly perceived a power shift away from the relative autonomy their departments had enjoyed. They preferred fragmentation and the political sleight-of-hand possible, where they were individually responsible for their plans, which could be rationalized and slipped through a largely uninformed review process. Second, and equally important, candidates for potential senior planning positions perceived that they were in high-risk, high-visibility posts that had a large potential for visible failure and conflict with other Ministry departments. Volunteers were not widely forthcoming, and prospective appointees from the outside, from the Planning Ministry, for example, were relatively easy to discredit because they did not offer credible health experience. Efforts to breathe life into the Planning Department remained largely illusionary throughout the period of the project.

B. Manager Development

Basic manpower planning requires fairly reliable and available information on job structure and personnel qualification: What are the job definitions? What is the stock of existing staff? and What inflows and outflows can be anticipated?

While this principle was understood by the senior Ministry staff, effective actions to improve the situation were consistently sidetracked. Two factors in particular contributed to this failure.

1. *Corruption in the transfer process.* Personnel transfers represented one of the few consistently important decision points where influence— either in terms of cash or debts of personal obligation—could readily be brought to bear with great impact on an individual's career. Posts varied widely in terms of social, economic, or personal development potential. This placed substantial power in the hands of the Personnel-Transfer Committee and the administrative office that served it. The experience of working intimately within the Ministry produced remarkably few suggestions of under-the-table dealings; the personnel-transfer process was a notable exception.

2. *Availability of posting information.* The prospect of improved organization and access to information on personnel qualifications and posts were presented and developed with the Personnel Department. The team's underlying assumption was that improved information *quality* would improve the *process* of personnel placement without necessarily disrupting tacitly acknowledged rules by which decisions were reached. This proved wrong. In the end, the personnel office staff was more afraid of the increased pressure they felt would be generated by widespread knowledge of the availability of desirable posts than they were attracted to the simplicity and order the proposed system changes would bring to their jobs.

The inability of the Ministry, with the team's assistance, to act effectively on personnel-planning issues leaves a major deficiency in Afghanistan's ability to pursue an effective health-development process. Programs are staffed ad hoc, and longer-range plans for the creation and use of new staff are built on very shaky foundations.

Chronology

1972	Preliminary project design Dr. Ibrahim Majid Seraj, Minister
July 1973	Mohammed Daoud seizes power, overthrows monarchy and proclaims Republic of Afghanistan with himhimself as President
August 1973	Dr. Sekandar appointed Minister of Public Health
September 1973	MSH team arrives in Kabul
December 1973	Drug-import analysis completed
1974	New AID health officer arrives (stays until 1979)
March 1974	MSH's initial analysis and workplan completed
October 1974	Parwan-Kapisa Pilot Project begins
March 1975	Auxiliary Nurse-Midwife (ANM) School opens
1975	New warehouse manual completed
April 1975	Basic Health Center manuals introduced
July 1975	Parwan-Kapisa survey completed
November 1975	MSH team member arrives (replaces original member)
February 1976	Basic Health Services' "twelve-province expansion" completed
March 1976	Dr. Abdul Omar appointed Minister of Public Health
April 1976	National implementation of Basic Health Center mobile training teams
August 1976	Three-province survey begins
October 1976	Three new MSH team members arrive; two leave (making a total of five team members)
October 1976	Basic Health Center manual evaluation
October 1976	Country health programming exercise (for 7-year plan) begins
1977	National generic drug law passed
February 1977	Three-province survey completed

March 1977	VHW manuals completed
April 1977	Basic Health Center training evalution
April 1977	VHW Program approved by Afghan cabinet
May 1977	First VHWs trained in Sarobi
June 1977	First *dais* trained in Girishk
June 1977	Girishk Regional Training Center opens
July 1977	AID evaluation of MSH project
August 1977	Baseline village survey in Jaghori completed
November 1977	Establishment of logistics coordinating office in Ministry of Public Health
January 1978	Home-visiting experiment completed
March 1978	Nationwide implementation of *Dai* program begins
March 1978	Establishment of Financial Analysis Office
April 1978	Coup overthrows Daoud; Democratic Republic of Afghanistan established
May 1978	Dr. Shah Wali appointed Minister of Public Health
July 1978	Logistics manual completed
August 1978	First nutrition rehabilitation/oral rehydration unit opened
March 1979	VHW Program suspended
May 1979	Health-education manual for Basic Health Centers completed
June 1979	MSH departs Afghanistan
December 1979	U.S.S.R. occupies Afghanistan

Glossary

Abbreviations

AHDS	Alternative Health Delivery System
AID	(United States) Agency for International Development
ANM	Auxiliary nurse-midwife
API	Avicenna Pharmaceutical Institute. This is the Afghan government's agency for drug import, manufacture, and control. It sells drugs to both governmental and private pharmacies, as well as to governmental health services. Formerly the General Medical Depot (GMD).
BHC	Basic Health Center
BHSD	Basic Health Services Department. This department, within the Ministry of Public Health, was responsible for Basic Health Centers, village health workers, and the *Dai* Training Program.
CHP	Country Health Programming. This is a comprehensive health-planning process promoted by the World Health Organization.
COP	Chief of party. This is a title used by USAID to designate the head of a contract team working in a specific country.
EPI	Expanded Program of Immunization
MCH	Maternal and child health
MOPH	Ministry of Public Health
MSH	Management Sciences for Health (The team, management team)
PHI	Public Health Institute
Team	The MSH management team
TEMO	Transport and Equipment Maintenance Organization. TEMO was an Afghan government agency,

assisted by UNICEF, responsible for MOPH vehicle and medical-equipment maintenance and repairs.

UNFPA   United Nations Fund for Population Activities

UNDP   United Nations Development Program

UNICEF   United Nations International Children's Fund

USAID   United States Agency for International Development.

VHW   Village health worker

WFP   World Food Program, a UNDP Activity of the FAO

WHO   World Health Organization

Farsi (Afghan Language) Words

Afghan   A person from Afghanistan

Afghani   An Afghani is the basic unit of currency in Afghanistan. In 1978 Afghanis, 100 was approximately equal to US$2.50.

atar   *Atars* are shopkeepers or sidewalk vendors who specialize in the sale of herbal medicines

dai   A *dai* is a traditional birth attendant. In addition to assisting at childbirth, this usually older woman is frequently consulted regarding other health problems of women and children.

dokhan   *Dokhans* are small village shops that sell a variety of essential items, frequently including medicines such as aspirin, vitamin C, and ointments.

dokhandar   A shopkeeper.

hakim   Sometimes called *hakimji*, these are traditional medical practitioners and are often Hindu. They use a combination of methods derived from both India and from the Greco-Arabic traditions.

jinns   *Jinns* is a folk classification for childhood deaths attributable to evil spirits with an attraction to the very young.

mullah   The *mullah* is an Islamic religious leader. In addition, he is frequently consulted to cure or prevent illness.

Pashtu   This is the second major language of Afghanistan.

Pashtun   A *Pashtun* is a *Pashtu*-speaking Afghan, usually from the southwestern and southern provinces.

Shekesta bande   This is the traditional bonesetter.

tawildar   The *tawildar* (*tavildar*) is a traditional position in Afghan commerce and government. His name may be translated as either storekeeper or trustee. He may be bonded and has custody of specified property or even money.

wolesmal   Multi-purpose rural-development worker employed by the Rural Development Department.

woleswal   The *woleswal* is appointed by the Interior Ministry to be head of all government services within a *woleswali*.

woleswali   This is the major subdivision or district of a province. There are about 180 *woleswalis* in Afghanistan.

Afghan Calendar

The calendar used in Afghanistan is one of two Islamic calendars that start with the flight of Muhammad from Mecca in A.D. 622. The Afghan calendar is a solar calendar that begins every year on the twenty-first of March. For the period of the Basic Health Services Project, the Afghan years are as follows:

Afghan Year	*Gregorian Calendar Equivalents*
1352	21 March 1973 to 20 March 1974
1353	21 March 1974 to 20 March 1975
1354	21 March 1975 to 20 March 1976
1355	21 March 1976 to 20 March 1977
1356	21 March 1977 to 20 March 1978
1357	21 March 1978 to 20 March 1979
1358	21 March 1979 to 20 March 1980

For convenience to most readers, the text uses the Gregorian calendar years.

List of MSH/Afghanistan Documents

20. Basic Health Center System, Plan of Operation, 1354–1356, August 1975
21. Preliminary Outline for National Rural Health System: Proposal for a Pilot Project (September 1975)
22. A Proposal for the Two-Stage Development of a Rural Health Logistics System, September 1975
23. Parwan BHC Pilot Project Evaluation Report Summary, March 1976
24. Draft: Proposal for Improving the World Food Program Project in Basic Health Centers, June 24, 1976
25. Country Health Programs Budget and Manpower Tables, November 1976
26. Ministry of Public Health, Basic Health Services Plan of Action for 1356 (March 1977–March 1978) November 1976
27. Draft: Afghan National Health Program, 1355–1361 December 30, 1976
28. Financial Analysis of Health Programs, Ministry of Public Health, Republic of Afghanistan, 2nd Draft, January 1977
29. Justification of 1356 Budget Request Increases, Ministry of Public Health, February 20, 1977
30. Evaluation of the Basic Health Services Manuals (Third Printing), March 1977
31. A Proposed Village Health Worker Program for the People of Afghanistan, March 23, 1977 (Primary Health Care through Village Health Workers)
32. Proposal for Girishk Regional Training/Health Center, March 1977
33. Field Manual for Village Health Workers, April 1977
34. Basic Health Center Manuals, Series 3, June 1977
35. Management Support for Rural and Family Health Services Project Status, March 1975 (MSH/B publication)
36. Basic Health Services Statistics, A Summary Analysis, September 1974
37. Project Request for UNFPA, National *Dai* Training Program, October 1977 (English only)
38. Report on the VHW Program, October 15, 1977
39. Financial Projections for the MOPH of the GOA, October 1977
40. Proposal for an Improved Drug Supply to BHCs, February 22, 1976
41. NM and ANM Output in Afghanistan, September 1977
42. *Dai* Training Curricula, 3rd Revision, October 1977
43. A Health Survey of Three Provinces of Afghanistan, November 1977
44. A Report on Personnel Information System, August 1978
45. A Report on Girishk Regional Training Center, August 1978
46. A Strategy for In-Country Management Training for the Ministry of Public Health, Draft, July 1978

References

Aarons, Audrey and Hawes, Hugh, with Juliet Gayton. *Child-to-Child.* London: MacMillan Press, Ltd., 1979.

American Public Health Association. *The State of the Art of Delivering Low Cost Health Services in Less Developed Countries: A Summary Study of 180 Projects.* Washington, D.C.: American Public Health Association, 1974.

Bernier, D.W., Bunge, F.M., Rintz, F.C., Shinn, R., Smith, H.H., and Teleki, S. *Area Handbook for Afghanistan.* Washington, D.C.: Government Printing Office, 1973.

Blumenhagen, Jeanne. *The Hazarajat Project.* Illinois: Medical Assistance Programs, Inc., 1971.

Blumenhagen, Rex V. and Blumenhagen, Jeanne. *Family Health Care: A Rural Health Care Delivery Scheme.* Illinois: Medical Assistance Programs, Inc., 1974.

Blumenhagen, Rex V., and Blumenhagen, Jeanne. *Final Report with Summary of Experience and Recommendations for a Health Care Delivery System.* Illinois: Medical Assistance Programs, Inc., 1974.

Briscoe, J. "The Role of Water Supply in Improving Health in Poor Countries (with special reference to Bangladesh)." *American Journal of Clinical Nutrition* 31 (1978): 2100–2113.

Bryant, John. *Health and the Developing World.* New York: Cornell University Press, 1969.

Cameron, Margaret and Yngre Hofvander. *Manual on Feeding Infants and Young Children.* New York: United Nations, 1976.

Clarke, J.C. "Survey of Venereal Diseases in Afghanistan." *WHO Bulletin* 2 (1950): 689–703.

Dupree, Louis. *Afghanistan.* Princeton: Princeton University Press, 1980.

Dupree, Louis. "Population Review, 1970: Afghanistan." *Field Staff Reports.* South Asia Series, American University Field Staff, 15, no. 1, 1971.

Feachem, R., Burn, E., Cairncross, S. et al. *Water, Health, and Development.* London: Tri-Med Books, 1978.

Fischer, L. *Afghanistan: Geomedical Monograph.* Geomedical Monograph Series, Regional Studies in Geographic Medicine. Berlin, Heidelberg, New York: SpringerVerlag, 1968.

Furnia, Arthur H. *Syncrisis: The Dynamics of Health, XXIV: Afghanistan.* U.S. Department of Health, Education, and Welfare: March 1978.

Ghosh, Shanti. *The Feeding and Care of Infants and Young Children.* New Delhi: Voluntary Health Association of India, August 1976.

Gish, O. and Walker, G. *Mobile Health Services.* London: Tri-Med Books, 1977.

Gordon, J.E., Behar, M., and Scrimshaw, N.S. "Acute Diarrheal Disease in Less Developed Countries: Three Methods for Prevention and Control." *WHO Bulletin* 31 (1964): 21–28.

Gregorian, Vartan. *The Emergence of Modern Afghanistan.* Stanford: Stanford University Press, 1969.

Haikal, Qadir. *Nursing and Midwifery in Aghanistan.* Nicosia: Regional Office for the Eastern Mediterranean, World Health Organization, 1970.

Hirschhorn, N., Lamstein, J.H., O'Connor, R.W., and Denny, K. "Logical Flow Diagrams in the Training of Health Workers." *Journal of Tropical Pediatrics and Environmental Child Health* April 1975.

Institute of Development Studies Research Reports. *Health Needs and Health Services in Rural Ghana.* Brighton, England: University of Sussex, 1978.

Kerr, Graham B., Macey, Anne, Hunte, Pam, Kamiab, Hassan, and Safi, Mahbouda. *Indigenous Fertility Regulation Methods in Afghanistan.* Afghan Demographic Studies, Afghan Family Guidance Association, Kabul, Afghanistan. Family Guidance Research Report, no. 8, April 1975.

Kerr, Graham B., Macey, Anne, Hunte, Pam, Kamiab, Hassan, and Safi, Mahbouda. *Afghan Family Guidance Clients and Their Husbands Compared with Non-Client Neighbors and Their Husbands.* Afghan Demographic Studies, Afghan Family Guidance Association, Kabul, Afghanistan. Family Guidance Research Report, no. 9, June 1975.

Kielmann, A.A. and McCord, C.M. "Home Treatment of Childhood Diarrhea in Punjab Villages." *Journal of Tropical Pediatrics and Environmental Child Health* 23 (1977): 197–201.

King, Maurice. *Medical Care in Developing Countries.* London: Oxford University Press, 1966.

King, Maurice H., King, Felicity M.A., Morley, David C., Burgess, H.J. Leslie, and Burgess, Ann P. *Nutrition for Developing Countries.* London: Oxford University Press, 1972.

Koppert, Joan. *Nutrition Rehabilitation: Its Practical Application.* London: Tri-Med Books, Ltd., 1977.

Macey, Ann, Hunte, Pam, and Kamiab, Hassan. *Indigenous Medical Practitioners in Afghanistan.* Afghan Demographic Studies, Afghan Family Guidance Association, Kabul, Afghanistan. Family Guidance Research Report, no. 13, June 1975.

Miazad, Rafiq. "Friend of Health." *World Health* May 1978, pp. 20–21.

Ministry of Health and Family Welfare, New Delhi, Government of India. *Manual for Community Health Worker.* October 1977.

Ministry of Planning, Kabul, Afghanistan. *First Seven Year Economic and Social Development Plan, 1355-1361, (March 1976-March 1983).* 1976.

Ministry of Public Health, Kabul, Afghanistan. *Afghan Journal of Public Health. passim.* 1975-1979.

Ministry of Public Health, Kabul, Afghanistan. *Infant and Early Childhood Mortality in Relation to Fertility Patterns, Report on an Ad-Hoc Survey in Greater Kabul, Afghanistan: 1972-1975.* World Health Organization, Regional Office for the Eastern Mediterranean, 1978.

Ministry of Public Health, Departments of Basic Health Services and Preventive Medicine, Democratic Republic of Afghanistan. "Primary Health Care in Afghanistan." *Assignment Children* no. 42 (April-June, 1978): 129-138.

Morley, David. *Paediatric Priorities in the Developing World.* London: Butterworth and Co., Ltd., 1973.

Newell, Kenneth W. *Health by the People.* World Health Organization, Geneva, Switzerland, 1975.

Newell, Richard S. *The Politics of Afghanistan.* Ithaca: Cornell University Press, 1972.

Preston, S.H., *Mortality Patterns in National Populations: With Special Reference to Recorded Causes of Death.* New York: Academic Press, 1976.

Puffer, R.R. and Serrano, C.V. *Patterns of Mortality in Childhood.* Washington, D.C.: Pan American Health Organization, 1973.

Rohde, Jon E., and Northrup, Robert S. "Therapy Begins at Home." New Developments in Pediatric Research, *International Congress Pediatrics* 15 (1977): 809-819.

Ronaghy, Hossain A. and Solter, Steven L. "Is the Chinese 'Barefoot Doctor' Exportable to Rural Iran." *The Lancet,* (29 June 1974) pp. 1331-1333.

Ronaghy, Hossain A., Najarzadeh, Ebrahim, Schwartz, Terry A., Russell, Sharon Stanton, Solter, Steven, and Zeighami, Bahram. "The Front Line Health Worker: Selection, Training, and Performance." *American Journal of Public Health* 66, no. 3 (March 1976): 273-277.

Rousselle, P.J., O'Connor, R.W., Hartman, A.F., Quick, J.D., and Bates, J.A. "Procurement and Use of Drugs: Managing the Process to Advantage." *New Developments in Vaginal Contraception* April 1979.

Schneider, R.E., Shiffman, M., and Faigenblum, J. "The Potential Effect of Water on Gastrointestinal Infections Prevalent in Developing Countries." *American Journal of Clinical Nutrition* 31 (1978): 2089-2099.

Scrimshaw, N.S., Taylor, C.E., and Gordon, J.E. "Interactions of Nutrition and Infection." *American Journal of Medical Sciences* 237 (1959): 367-403.

Smith, Richard A. (ed.). *Manpower and Primary Health Care: Guidelines for Improving/Expanding Health Service Coverage in Developing Countries.* Honolulu: University Press of Honolulu, 1978.

State University of New York, Buffalo, New York. *National Demographic and Family Guidance Survey of the Settled Population of Afghanistan.* Vols. 1 and 2, 1975.

Stone, Russell A. and Kerr, Graham B. *Afghan Pharmacists: Their Knowledge and Attitude Towards Family Guidance.* Afghan Demographic Studies, Afghan Family Guidance Association, Kabul, Afghanistan, Family Guidance Research Report, no. 4, June 1973.

Suyadi, A., Sadjimin, T., Rohde, Jon E. "Primary Care in the Village: An Approach to Village Self-Help Health Programmes." *Tropical Doctor* 7 (1977): 123–128.

Taylor, C.E., Kielmann, A.A., Parker, R.L., et al. *Malnutrition, Infection, Growth, and Development: The Narangwal Experience, Final Report.* Washington, D.C.: World Bank, 1978.

Toynbee, A.J. *Between Oxus and Jumma.* New York: Oxford University Press, 1961.

United States Agency for International Development, Kabul, Afghanistan. *Health Sector Assessment and Strategy,* 1978.

United States Agency for International Development, Kabul, Afghanistan. *Project Paper: Basic Health Services, Afghanistan,* 1978.

Verderese, Maria de Lourdes and Tumbull, Lily M. *The Traditional Birth Attendant in Maternal and Child Health and Family Planning: A Guide to Her Training and Utilization.* World Health Organization, Geneva, Switzerland, 1975. (WHO Offset Publication, no. 18).

Werner, David. *Where There Is No Doctor: A Village Health Care Handbook.* Palo Alto, California: The Hesperian Foundation, 1977.

World Health Organization. *Declaration of Alma Ata.* (Report on the International Conference on Primary Health Care, Alma Ata, USSR, 6–12 September 1978).

Index

Index

Management Sciences for Health

Management Sciences for Health (MSH) was established in 1971 as an independent foundation that works worldwide to promote the practical application of management techniques in health and to increase knowledge in the field. Internationally, MSH has worked with host governments on the development and implementation of health services in more than thirty countries in Asia, Africa, and Latin America, often sponsored by international and bilateral donor agencies or directly by the host-country institutions.

Domestically, MSH is involved in the development, testing, and implementation of consumer-health-education strategies for personal health promotion in school, community, and workplace settings.

The multinational professional staff of MSH includes specialists in management, medicine, statistics, epidemiology, education, computer and social sciences, and public health.

The Management Team

The Field Team

Chiefs of Party
Terrence V. O'Connor, 1973–1976
Henry R. Norman, 1976–1978
Jerry M. Russell, 1978–1979

Administrative Assistants
Stephanie Sediqzad
Carol Safi
Lorna Hoge Taraki

Field Staff
Steven J. Fabricant, 1973–1975
Richard Moore, 1973–1976
Ernst L. Lauridsen, 1974–1976
Peter N. Cross, 1975–1979
Jerry M. Russell, 1976–1978
Steven L. Solter, 1976–1979
John W. LeSar, 1977–1979
James Bates, 1978–1979

Field Consultants
Anne Kesterton, 1975
Paul Kesterton, 1974–1976
Lynette Russell, 1976
Kathy LeSar, 1978–1979

The Home Office

Director of International Programs   *Administrative Assistants*

Peter J. Rouselle   Judy Mason, 1973–1975
                                      Donna Vincent, 1976–1978
                                      Patricia McCarthy, 1978–1979

Project Director

Ronald W. O'Connor, 1973–1979

Project Coordinators

Kevin M. Denny, 1973–1976
Terrence V. O'Connor, 1976–1978
A. Frederick Hartman, 1978–1979

About the Contributors

James Bates was a management consultant concerned primarily with logistics systems for the Afghan Ministry of Health. He was educated at the University of Wisconsin and received the masters degree with a concentration in public administration in Muslim societies. He worked in Afghanistan for the Peace Corps and as a staff associate at Management Sciences for Health. Mr. Bates is currently working with Latin American and Middle Eastern governments on public-health management.

Peter N. Cross was educated at the California Institute of Technology and did doctoral work at the Graduate School of Public and International Affairs at the University of Pittsburgh. Mr. Cross worked in Nepal on educational and agricultural development and with the Afghan Ministry of Health on financial planning and management of village health programs.

John W. LeSar M.D. received undergraduate and medical training at Ohio State University and completed a residency in international health at Johns Hopkins University. After 2 years as director of evaluation for the Medex Program at the University of Hawaii, Dr. LeSar joined the Management Sciences for Health team in Kabul, coordinating the Basic Health Services and *Dai* Training Programs. He is currently on leave from Management Sciences for Health while acting as the Health, Population, and Nutrition Officer for U.S. Agency for International Development in India.

Henry Norman, a lawyer by training and an international-development worker by experience, is currently executive director of Volunteers in Technical Assistance (VITA). Mr Norman served as an early Peace Corps country director in Africa and as chief of party in Afghanistan, with additional technical responsibilities for basic health-service development.

Jerry M. Russell received doctoral training in public-health administration at the University of North Carolina at Chapel Hill. He has worked with voluntary Health agencies in India, as the administrative director for the International Postpartum Family Planning Program of the Population Council, and as the last chief of party for the Management Sciences for Health team in Afghanistan. He is currently health, population, and nutrition officer for Haiti with U.S. Agency for International Development.

Steven L. Solter, M.D., received undergraduate and medical training at the University of California at Berkeley and Stanford University, completed a residency in international health at Johns Hopkins University, and served as an epidemic intelligence service officer at the Center for Disease Control. Dr. Solter worked on the early phases of village health-worker training in

Shiraz, Iran, and was the principal consultant to the Afghan government in its development of village-based health workers. He is currently coordinating the Nepal Integrated Rural Health Services Project and consulting on rural health development in Asia and the Middle East.

Lorna Hoge Taraki was administrative officer for the Management Sciences for Health team in Afghanistan and previously held similar positions with the Afghan Demographic Studies Program and the Public Administration Service during more than 15 years in Afghanistan.

Stephen C. Thomas, M.D. is an obstetrician-gynecologist who worked for many years with the Kaiser Permanente Medical Group prior to earning the masters degree in public health at the University of Michigan and entering the international-health field. Dr. Thomas is currently working in Syria as health program officer with AID.

About the Editor

Ronald W. O'Connor, M.D., was graduated from Yale University and completed medical training at the College of Physicians and Surgeons, Columbia University. While at Columbia he spent a year in Asia studying medical education and was a fellow at the School of International Affairs. Following work as epidemic intelligence service officer at the Center for Disease Control, he received the master's degrees in public health from Harvard University and in management from the Massachusetts Institute of Technology. He founded Management Sciences for Health while at M.I.T. and has been a director since.

Aside from international health interests, he is working on curricula to form health-habits among primary- and secondary-school children.